WINE AND FOOD HANDBOOK

Aide-Mémoire for the sommelier and the waiter

Revised and ~~edited~~ by
John Cousins and Cailein Gillespie

The Food and Beverage Training Company, London
The Scottish Hotel School, Glasgow

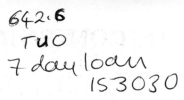

642.6
TUO
7 day loan
153030

Orders: please contact Bookpoint Ltd, 130 Milton Park, Abingdon, Oxon
OX14 4SB. Telephone: (44) 01235 827720. Fax: (44) 01235 400454. Lines
are open from 9.00–5.00, Monday to Saturday, with a 24-hour message
answering service. You can also order through our website
www.hoddereducation.co.uk

British Library Cataloguing in Publication Data
A catalogue record for this title is available from the British Library

ISBN: 978 0 340 84852 4

First published in 1977
Impression number   10 9 8 7 6
Year   2007

Cover photo from Photodisc
Typeset by Dorchester Typesetting Group Ltd
Printed in Great Britain for Hodder Arnold, an imprint of Hodder
Education and a member of the Hodder Headline Group, an Hachette
Livre UK Company, 338 Euston Road, London NW1 3BH by
CPI Antony Rowe Limited

CONTENTS

ACKNOWLEDGEMENTS

The preparation of the second edition of the *Wine and Food Handbook* has drawn upon a variety of experience and literature. We would like to express our thanks to those who have given their assistance and support in the revision of this text. In preparing this new edition we would specifically like to thank:

Andrew Durkan, author and consultant, formally of Ealing College, London; Professor David Foskett, author, consultant and Associate Dean at the London School of Tourism, Hospitality and Leisure, Ealing; Dennis Lillicrap, consultant, author and trainer in food and beverage service; Andrew Morgan, Food and Beverage Services Manager, and the team at Restaurant One-O-One, Knightsbridge, London; Robert Smith, Head of Food and Beverage Service at the Birmingham College of Food, Tourism and Creative Studies, and in particular Samuel Salvisberg, Senior Vice-President, Ecole hôtelière de Lausanne, Switzerland for providing the tribute to Conrad Tuor given on page 6.

In preparing this new edition we have also adapted material from some of our own publications, including:

- *The Beverage Book*, Durkan, A. and Cousins, J., Hodder and Stoughton, London, 1995
- *Customer Service Skills CD-ROM*, Gillespie, C., Butterworth–Heinemann, Oxford, 2001
- *European Gastronomy Into the 21st Century*, Gillespie, C., (Contributing Editor Cousins J.), Butterworth–Heinemann, Oxford, 2001
- *Food and Beverage Management Mediabase*, Gillespie, C., Butterworth–Heinemann, Oxford, 2001
- *Food and Beverage Service*, 6th Edition, Lillicrap D., Cousins, J. and Smith, R., Hodder and Stoughton, London, 2002
- *Food and Beverage Management*, 2nd Edition, Cousins J., Foskett D. and Gillespie C., Pearson Education, Harlow, 2002
- *The Student Guide to Food and Drink*, Cousins, J. and Durkan, A., Hodder and Stoughton, 1992

- *Teach Yourself Wine Appreciation*, Durkan, A. and Cousins, J., Hodder and Stoughton, 1995.

Other sources of reference, which have been consulted, include:

- *Larousse Encyclopaedia of Wine*, Larousse International, Hammersmith, 2001
- *Larousse Gastronomique*, Hamlyn, London, 2001
- *Le Répertoire de la Cuisine,* 17th Edition, Saulnier, L., Leon Jaeggi & Sons Ltd, Middlesex, 1985
- *The Oxford Companion to Wine*, Robinson, J., Oxford University Press, Oxford, 1999
- *Practical Cookery*, 9th Edition, Ceserani, V., Kinton, R. and Foskett, D., Hodder and Stoughton, London, 2000
- *Wine with Food:* the ultimate guide to matching wine with food for every occasion, Simon, J., Mitchell Beazley, London, 1999.

MR. CONRAD TUOR

Mr. Tuor entered the Ecole hôtelière de Lausanne as a member of its Faculty on April 1st, 1948. He introduced and contributed a new frame of mind to this institution, which in those days was still located in town on Avenue de Cour. This frame of mind was mainly made up of an unfailing love for one's trade, a vocation, a faultless conscientiousness and most of all a true pleasure in training others.

Being a man experienced in the industry, Mr. Tuor always felt the need to keep in touch with customers and enjoyed an impeccable professional standing. He very soon wanted to confront the theory he was teaching at the School with industrial practice. Therefore, he first expressed his educational wish, and very soon enabled his students, to move on to real-life situations. Thus he broke new ground setting up an external service, which eventually resulted in nearly 7,000 contracts ranging from the most unpretentious banquet to major events gathering over four thousand guests.

In 1948 Mr. Tuor wrote the book entitled *L'aide-mémoire du sommelier*. He designed it first of all as a practical tool, comprehensive and easy to refer to. *"I wrote this book when I was still bubbling over with the passion of everyday practice, before I became "contaminated" with theory"*, he used to say jokingly.

In February 1979, after working for 31 years as a lecturer teaching service courses, Mr. Tuor officially took his leave of the School. With great wisdom and clear-sightedness, he said to the audience who had gathered to pay tribute to him:

> *"Over the past decade, the School underwent essential and necessary changes. Nevertheless it has not discarded two basic requirements, which are particularly dear to me: behaviour and promptness. These two requirements are the very symbols of our tradition and continuity. They strike me as being two virtues vital to this wonderful trade, which still needs to undergo improvements without however betraying the principles that built up and nourished its glorious past".*

Mr. Tuor passed away on July 27, 2000.

Samuel Salvisberg, Senior Vice-President, Ecole hôtelière de Lausanne, 27 June 2002

PREFACE

In revising and editing this edition of the *Wine and Food Handbook* we acknowledge the achievements of the late Conrad Tuor who was the Maître d'Hôtel Professor, The Hotel School, Lausanne, Switzerland. It was through his desire to contribute to learning in this great profession, that the original Swiss edition was created. It was used for many years in top-class hotels, restaurants and hotel schools throughout the world, and also by anyone interested in good living. The English edition, was first published in 1977, and respected the original intentions of Conrad Tuor. It is the English edition that has provided the inspiration for this revision of Conrad Tuor's classic work.

The overall aim has been to preserve the original intention and orientation of the book, with the title of the new edition of the book now given in full as: *Wine and Food Handbook—Aide-Mémoire for the sommelier and the waiter*. In acknowledgement of the work of Conrad Tuor, and to honour his name, we proposed from the start that the front cover should carry the name of Conrad Tuor only.

The new edition is presented in three key parts. These are:

Part 1 Service—which considers various aspects of food and beverage service

Part 2 Wine and other drinks—which covers wine and other alcoholic and non-alcoholic bar drinks, and cigars

Part 3 Cuisine, Lay-Ups and Accompaniments—which covers a range of menu courses, dishes and the service of them

These three parts are then supported by four listings:

- **Cocktails and mixed drinks listing**
- **Glossary of some cuisine and service terms**
- **The origin of some classical menu terms**
- **Vocabulary (French, German and English)**

The specific aims of the new edition of the book are to:

- meet the needs of students and working sommeliers and waiters who are seeking a quick reference guide to aspects of European food, wines and other drinks and the service of them;

- be of value to anyone interested in good food, wine and other drinks and good living, and to

- encourage curiosity and fascination, a desire for discovery through investigation and experience, and ultimately fulfilment as industry professionals and as gastronomes.

It has also been our intention, in preparing this text, to provide a new edition worthy of the original.

John Cousins and Cailein Gillespie, August 2002

FOOD AND BEVERAGE SERVICE

What is food and beverage service?

Food and beverage service is the essential link between the menu, beverages and other services on offer in an establishment and the customers. People working in food and beverage service are the main point of contact between customers and an establishment. It is an important role in a noble profession, with increasing National and International status. Skills and knowledge, and therefore careers, are transferable between establishments, sectors and throughout the world.

- **Food** can include a wide range of styles and cuisine types. These can be by country, e.g. traditional British or Italian, by type of cuisine e.g. oriental or aiming for a particular speciality such as fish, vegetarian or health food.

- **Beverages** include all alcoholic and non-alcoholic drinks. Alcoholic beverages include wines and all other types of alcoholic drink such as cocktails, beers and ciders, spirits and liqueurs. Non-alcoholic beverages include bar beverages such as mineral waters, juices, squashes and aerated waters, as well as tea, coffee, chocolate, milk and milk drinks and also proprietary drinks.

For a particular food and beverage (or foodservice) operation the choice as to how the food and beverage service is designed, planned, undertaken and controlled is made by taking account of various organisational variables. These variables include:

- customer needs
- level of customer demand
- the type and style of the food and beverage operation
- the nature of the customers (non-captive, captive or semi-captive)
- prices to be charged

- production process
- volume of demand
- volume of throughput
- space available
- availability of staff
- opening hours
- booking requirements
- payment requirements
- legal requirements.

Key staff requirements

For food and beverage service staff the four key requirements are:

1 Sound product knowledge;

2 Competent technical skills;

3 Well developed social skills; and

4 The ability to work as part of a team.

Whilst there have been changes in food and beverage service, with less emphasis on the high level technical skills being seen in some sectors, these four key requirements remain for all staff. However the emphasis on these key requirements varies according to the type of establishment and the particular service methods being used.

Key personal attributes of staff include having high standards of personal grooming, integrity, honesty, respect and professionalism, as well as being able to work hygienically and safely.

Types of food and beverage operations

Food and beverage service in its various forms is found, for instance, in various types of restaurants (e.g. first class, destination, bistros, brasseries, gastrodomes, coffee-shops, ethnic and themed), cafés, cafeterias, take-aways, canteens, function rooms, and in lounge and room service for hotel guests. There are also many types of business sector such as hotels, independent and chain restaurants, popular catering, pubs and wine bars, fast food, leisure attractions and banqueting. There are also sectors where food and beverages are provided as part of another business. These include transport catering, welfare, clubs, education, industrial feeding and the forces. In many cases the same type of operation, such as a table service restaurant, may be found in a wide variety of sectors.

Customer needs

The reasons for eating out vary. It could simply be having to eat out because the person is unable to return home or because the person is celebrating some special occasion such as a birthday. However the same people can have different needs at different times. In other words, it is important to consider the needs people have rather than the type of people that they are. This is because, for example, the person on business during a weekday can also be the family adult at the weekend, a conference delegate on another occasion and a traveller on the motorway on another. Needs that people have can be summarised as:

- Physiological needs, e.g. to satisfy hunger and thirst, or to satisfy the need for special foods.
- Economic needs, e.g. staying within a certain budget, wanting good value, a convenient location or fast service.
- Social needs, e.g. being out with friends, business colleagues or attending special functions such as weddings.
- Psychological needs, e.g. responding to advertising, wanting to try something new, fulfilling life-style needs or satisfying or fulfilling the need for self-esteem.
- Convenience needs, for example it may not be possible to return home or the desire may be there for someone else to prepare, serve and wash up.

The meal experience

Any decision to eat out takes account of the customers' needs and also what type of experience is to be undertaken. A number of factors influence this decision. These factors are often referred to as the meal experience factors, which are summarised below.

The food and beverages on offer

This includes the range of foods and beverages, choice, availability, flexibility for special orders and the quality of the food and beverages.

Level of service

Depending on the needs people have at the time, the level of service sought will be appropriate to these needs. For example, a romantic night out may call for a quiet table in a top-end restaurant, whereas a group of young friends might be seeking more informal service. This factor also takes into account services such as booking and account facilities, acceptance of credit cards and also the reliability of the operation's product.

Level of cleanliness and hygiene

This relates to the premises, equipment and staff. Over the last few years this factor has increased in importance in the customers' minds. The recent media focus on food production and the risks involved in buying food have heightened awareness of health and hygiene aspects.

Perceived value for money and price

Customers have perceptions of the amount they are prepared to spend and relate these to differing types of establishments and operations. There is also a relationship between price, (the amount required), cost (taking account of other costs such as travel, the cost of not going somewhere else, potential disappointment or cost of being made to feel embarrassed), value (perceived importance) and worth (perceived significance). Good value is only where worth exceeds costs.

Atmosphere of the establishment

This factor takes account of issues such as: design, decor, lighting, heating, furnishings, acoustics and noise levels, the other customers, the staff and the attitude of the staff.

Food and beverage service methods

Food and beverage service was traditionally seen primarily as a delivery system. However, food and beverage service actually consists of two separate systems, which are operating at the same time. These are:

- **The service sequence**—which is primarily concerned with the delivery of food and beverages to the customer
- **Customer processes**—which is concerned with the experience the customer undertakes

The service sequence

The service sequence is essentially the bridge between the production system, beverage provision and the customer process (or experience). The service sequence consists of seven stages. These are:

1 preparation for service
2 taking food and beverage orders
3 the serving of food and beverages
4 billing
5 clearing
6 dishwashing
7 clearing following service

For each of these seven stages, there are a variety of alternative ways of carrying them out.

Customer processes

The customer receiving the food and beverage product is required to undertake or observe certain requirements—this is the customer process. In food and beverage operations there are five basic processes. These are:

1 **Table service**—where the customer is served at a laid table. This type of service, which includes waiter service and bar counter service, is found in restaurants, cafés and in banqueting.

2 **Self-service**—where the customer is required to help him or herself from a buffet or counter. This type of service can be found in cafeterias and canteens.

3 **Assisted service**—where the customer is served part of the meal at a table and is required to obtain part through self-service from some form of display or buffet. This type of service is found in 'carvery'

type operations and is often used for meals such as breakfast in hotels.

4   **Single point service**—where the customer orders, pays and receives the food and beverages for instance at a counter, at a bar in licensed premises, in a fast-food operation, or at a vending machine.

5   **Specialised** service (or service *in situ*)—where the food and drink is taken to where the customer is. This includes tray service in hospitals and aircraft, trolley service, home delivery, lounge and room service.

In the first four of these customer processes, the customer comes to where the food and beverage service is offered and the service is provided in areas primarily designed for the purpose. However, in the fifth customer process the service is provided in another location and where the area is not primarily designed for the purpose. All modern food and beverage service methods can be grouped under these five customer processes.

For table service, the different types of waiter service are	
Silver/English Service	Presentation and service of food to a customer by waiting staff from a food flat or dish.
Family Service	Main courses plated and with vegetables, placed in multi-portion dishes on tables for customers to help themselves. Any sauces are usually offered
Plated/American service	Service of pre-plated foods to customers, now widely used in many establishments and in banqueting
Butler/French Service	Presentation of food individually to customers by food service staff for customers to serve themselves.
Russian Service	Table laid with food for customers to help themselves. (Also sometimes confusingly used to indicate Guéridon or Butler service).
Guéridon Service	Food served onto customer's plate at a side table or from a trolley. Also may include carving, cooking and flambé dishes, preparation of salads and dressings.

Job roles

There are a wide variety of roles within food and beverage service. These roles include:

- food and beverage manager/food service manager
- restaurant manager/restaurant supervisor
- head waiter/supervisor
- station head waiter/section supervisor
- station/section waiter
- junior waiter (commis, apprentices, busboys or busgirls)

Specialist staff roles include lounge service staff, room service staff, buffet and counter staff, food service assistants, bar staff, wine service staff in restaurants, wine butlers/wine waiter/sommelier, function and banqueting staff and cashiers.

However, in food and beverage service most of the basic skills required are transferable to any type of operation. For example, carrying plates, trays, glasses and cutlery, carving skills, beverage service skills are broadly similar wherever they are carried out. The variation is in the application of these skills, which is usually governed by the requirements of the particular establishment.

MENUS

Menus may be divided into two classes:

- **à la carte** (from the card) with dishes separately priced
- **table d'hôte** (table of the host) an inclusive price for the whole meal or for a specified number of courses e.g. any two or any four courses. There are, however, usually choices within each course.

Brasserie, coffee shop and popular catering menus are limited forms of à la carte menus with all the dishes listed and priced separately. Other menu terms used are **carte du jour** (literally card of the day)—which is usually a fixed meal with one or more courses for a set price. A **prix fixe** (fixed price) menu is similar. Sometimes the price of the meal also includes wine or other drinks.

Classic European menu sequence

Over the last 100 or so years the sequence of the European menu has taken on a classical format or order of dishes. This is used to layout menus as well as to indicate the order of the various courses. The sequence is:

1 Hors-d'oeuvres
2 Soups (potages)
3 Egg dishes (œufs)
4 Pasta and rice (farineux)
5 Fish (poisson)
6 Entrée (small, well garnished dishes)
7 Sorbet
8 Relevé (main roasts, larger joints)
9 Roast (rôti) (game or poultry dishes)
10 Vegetables (legumes)
11 Salad (salade)
12 Cold Buffet (buffet froid)
13 Cheese (fromage)
14 Sweets (entremets)
15 Savoury (savoureaux)
16 Fruit (dessert)

In addition, it is common for beverages (coffee, tea etc) to be served at the end of the meal. These are not usually counted as a course. Thus, if a meal is quoted as having four courses, this must mean that there are four food courses and that the beverages are in addition to these.

The menu sequence was, and is, based on a logical process of taste sensations and provides the guide for the compilation of both à la carte and table d'hôte menus. The sequence is also used as a guide for the compilation and the determination of the order of the courses for function and special party menus. Its use is evident in many examples of modern European menus, although the actual number of courses on a menu, and dishes within each course, will depend on the size and class of the establishment. It is also common for a number of courses to be grouped together. At its most simple this might comprise:

- starters—courses 1 to 4
- main courses—courses 5,6 and 8 to 12
- afters—courses 13 to 16
- beverages

The modern classic European menu sequence is derived from traditional European (mainly Franco–Russian, Swiss and English) cuisine and service influences. The menu structure and menu sequence can change considerably within the various world cuisines. Additionally, menu terms also vary, for instance in the USA a main course is commonly called an entrée and sweets commonly called dessert. The term dessert is also now becoming more commonly used to denote sweets generally. Also, although this sequence shows the cheese course after the main course and before the sweet course, it was common in Britain for the sweet to be offered before the cheese course: in the UK either sequence may still be found.

Breakfast

The four main types of breakfast are:

- **Café/thé simple:** Only coffee or tea are served (nothing to eat)
- **Café/thé complet:** Refers to Continental breakfast with coffee or tea
- **Continental breakfast:** Traditionally consisted of rolls and coffee. Nowadays it is not uncommon to find a Continental breakfast menu with a broader range of items such as cheese, ham, and fruit
- **Full breakfast:** Consists of two to eight courses and includes any of the items shown on page 19. Sometimes called English Breakfast or American Breakfast.

Examples of breakfast menu items

Juices	Orange, pineapple, grapefruit, tomato, prune, carrot, apple
Fresh and stewed fruit	Melon, strawberries, orange segments, grapefruit (half or segments), pineapple, apricots, peaches, mango, paw paw, lychees, figs, prunes (fresh and stewed)
Cereals	Cornflakes, 'Weetabix', 'Special K', 'Alpen', muesli, bran flakes, 'Rice Krispies', porridge
Yoghurts	Natural and fruit, regular and low fat
Fish	Fried or grilled kippers, poached smoked haddock (sometimes with poached eggs), grilled herring, fried or grilled plaice, fried or grilled sole, Kedgeree, smoked fish (sometimes including dishes like smoked salmon with scrambled eggs), marinated fish such as gravedlax
Eggs	Fried, poached, scrambled, boiled, plain or savoury filled omelette, Eggs Benedict
Meats	Bacon in various styles, various sausages, kidney, steak, gammon
Potatoes and vegetables	Hash browns, sauté potatoes, home fries, mushrooms, baked beans, fresh or grilled tomato
Pancakes and waffles	Regular pancakes or waffles, with maple syrup or other toppings, blueberry pancakes, wholemeal pancakes, griddle cakes
Cold Buffet	Hams, tongue, chicken, smoked cold meats, salamis, cheeses (often accompanied by fresh salad items)
Bread items	Toast, rolls, croissants, brioches, crisp breads, plain sliced white or brown bread, Danish pastries, American muffins, English muffins, spiced scones, tea cakes, doughnuts
Preserves	Jams, marmalade, honey
Beverages	Teas, coffees (including decaffeinated), chocolate, tisanes, proprietary beverages, milk, mineral waters

Breakfast may be served in guest apartments as room service, in lounges, and also in restaurants with either full table service or with assisted service supported by buffet displays. The change towards buffet style of service for breakfast has also increased the range of foods on offer. The buffet can be used for any type of breakfast with the most extensive often called American Buffet Breakfast. Examples of the full range of menu items that may be found are shown on page 19. Buffet breakfast menus are also often priced and offered at three main levels:

1 Continental—including juices, bread items and beverages

2 Cold Buffet—including those of continental breakfast plus selection from the cold items from the buffet

3 Full Breakfast—full selection from the buffet including hot cooked items

Afternoon tea

Afternoon tea may be classified into the two main types:

■ Full afternoon tea

■ High tea

The main difference between the two is that high tea is a more substantial meal, including main course items such as grills, toasted snacks, fish and meat dishes, cold sweets and ices, in addition to the afternoon tea fare. The meat dishes frequently include pies and the fish dishes are usually fried. Vegetables and fried potatoes are included with some of the hot dishes. An example of a full afternoon tea menu is given on page 21. The items are usually served in the order listed, and beverages are served first.

Afternoon tea may be served in guest apartments as room service, in lounges and also in restaurants with either full table service or with assisted service supported by buffet displays.

Menu Influences

Knowledge about the product is at the core of successful food and beverage service. This knowledge enables the server to advise the customer of the content, the methods used in making the dishes and also

Example of afternoon tea menu items	
Beverages	Variety of teas, coffee (including decaffeinated), chocolate, tisanes, proprietary beverages, milk, mineral waters
Assorted tea sandwiches	Smoked salmon, sardine, cucumber, egg and cress, egg and tomato, ham
Toasted items	Hot buttered toast, crumpets, teacakes, English muffin
Bread items	White, brown and fruit breads
Sweet items	Scones, assorted tea cakes, sliced gateaux, various pastries
Preserves	Various jams and preserves and honey

to ensure that the customer is provided with an appropriate lay-up, service and the correct accompaniments. Customer needs are also being influenced by healthy options, special diets, and cultural and religious influences.

The relationship between health and eating

Customers are increasingly looking for choice and are requiring specific information on methods of cooking, e.g. frying, low fat, low salt etc., which will enable them to achieve a balanced diet.

Also, the desire for healthier eating has led to product changes—alternatives to butter, such as Flora are often provided and frequently bread is not buttered in advance thereby allowing the customer to choose his or her requirements. In addition, the availability of lower fat milks, non-dairy creamers and non-sugar sweeteners is now standard.

Customers are also becoming increasingly interested in food hygiene and food safety generally. There are also particular reactions to developments in food technology such as irradiation and genetically modified organisms and how these technologies are being used. Some customers are seeking to avoid these foods and some operations are already using the avoidance of these foods as a marketing feature. The use of organic foods is being promoted in a similar way.

Special diets

There are a variety of medical conditions, including allergies, which affect customer choices, and which are more common than was generally understood. Special diets for customers may be as a result of:

Allergies to food items such as gluten in wheat rye and barley (known as coeliac), peanuts and their derivatives, sesame seeds and other nuts such as cashew, pecan, brazil and walnuts, as well as milk, fish, shellfish and eggs.

Diabetes (inability of the body to control the level of glucose within the blood) where the customer may be looking for low cholesterol food and the avoidance of high sugar dishes.

Low cholesterol diets where the customer will be looking for dishes that include polyunsaturated fats or limited quantities of animal fats. Dishes might include lean poached or grilled meats and fish, fruit and vegetables and low fat milk, cheese and yoghurt.

Low sodium/salt diets where the customer is seeking dishes that include low sodium/salt foods and cooking with very limited or no use of salt.

Cultural and religious influences

Various cultures and faiths have differing requirements with regard to the dishes/ingredients that may be consumed and often these requirements also cover preparation methods, cooking procedures and the equipment used. Examples of these are:

Hindus who do not eat beef and rarely pork, with some not eating any other meats, fish or eggs, and may be seeking cheese, milk and vegetarian dishes.

Jews who seek to consume only 'clean' (kosher) animals and therefore will not accept dishes of pork or pork products, shellfish or animal fats and gelatine from beasts considered to be unclean or not slaughtered according to the prescribed manner. There are also restrictions placed on methods of preparation and cookery and also the preparation and eating of meat and dairy products at the same meal is not allowed.

Muslims who will not eat meat offal or animal fat unless it is 'halal' (lawful, as required under Islamic Dietary Law) meat.

Sikhs who will not eat beef or pork with some keeping to a vegetarian diet. Others may eat fish, mutton, cheese and eggs. Sikhs will not eat 'halal' meat.

Roman Catholics where although restrictions on diet are now very limited many will not eat meats on Ash Wednesday or Good Friday, and some will not eat meat on Fridays.

Vegetarianism

Vegetarianism may derive from cultural, religious, moral or physiological considerations. The various forms of vegetarianism may be summarised as:

Vegetarians: semi (or demi) who will not eat red meats, or all meats other than poultry, or all meats. These customers will be looking for dishes that include fish and may include dairy produce and other animal products.

Vegetarians: lacto-ovo who will not eat all meat, fish, poultry but may eat milk, milk products and eggs.

Vegetarians: lacto who will not eat all meat, fish, and poultry but may eat milk and milk products.

Vegans who will not eat any foods of animal origin. These customers will be looking for dishes mainly consisting of vegetables, vegetable oils, cereals, nuts, fruits and seeds.

Fruitarians, a more restricted form of vegetarianism, and these customers will not eat foods of animal origin or any pulses and cereals. These customers may be seeking dishes consisting of mainly raw and dried fruit, nuts, honey and olive oil.

SOME SERVICE CONVENTIONS

Use standard lay-ups
Indicates the type of meals being taken, the sequence of the courses and also what stage customers are at within a meal.

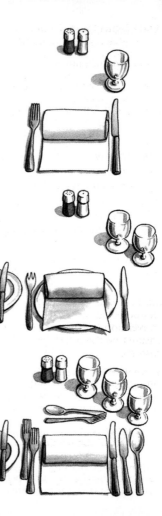

Classic, or basic lay-up: fish knife and fork or joint knife and fork and napkin, together with glassware and salt and pepper. Additional flatware and cutlery items are laid before each course is served.

À la carte lay-up: fish knife and fork and a fish plate, napkin and side plate and side knife, together with glassware and salt and pepper. Additional flatware and cutlery items are laid before each course is served.

Table d'hote lay-up: soup spoon, fish knife and fork, joint knife and fork and sweet spoon and fork, napkin and side plate and side knife, together with glassware and salt and pepper. Tableware for the whole meal is adjusted once the order has been taken.

Place items low to high
Lower items should be placed nearer the guest and taller items behind or to the side of these. Makes items easily accessible by the guest and can also avoid accidents.

Place items according to the guests position at the table
Items placed on a table should be within reach of the guest and also so that handles etc. are set for the guests' convenience.

Look for indications of special needs
Look out for, and be prepared to deal with, people with sight, hearing, speech, mobility and language difficulties. Also be able to deal with the needs of children.

Use order notation techniques
Helps with identifying, for any server, which member of a party is having what items of food or drink.

Take food, wine and drink orders through hosts
This is common courtesy—agreement needs to be obtained for any items that are to be served. For larger parties the orders may be taken individually, but it is useful to confirm what has actually been ordered with the host as this may save any disagreements later.

Start service from the right hand side of the host, with the host last
Honoured guests are usually seated on the right of a host. Also convention is to serve a table by moving anticlockwise to each guest to ensure that the serving staff are walking forwards to serve the next customer.

Serve women first
Often done if it does not slow the service. Particular care needs to be taken so as not to confuse things when the host is a woman. A host of either gender is still the host and should always be served last.

Place foods on the plate consistently
For service of the whole main course onto a joint plate, place the main item at the 6 o'clock position with potatoes served next at the 10 past 2 position and vegetables last at the 10 to 2 position (this also follows the UK Royal National Institute for the Blind (RNIB) recommendations). For

main courses with potatoes and vegetables and/or salads served on a separate plate or crescent, the main item is placed in the centre of the main plate and the separate plate or crescent of potatoes and vegetables and/or side salad to the left of this.

Silver serve food from the left-hand side of a guest
Ensures that the service dish is nearer the plate for ease of service and to prevent food being spilt onto the customer; customers can more easily see the food being served, and make choices if necessary, and service staff are also able to see and control what they are doing.

Use separate service gear for different food items
This should be standard. It avoids different food items not being transferred from one dish or plate to another and avoids food being messy on the guests' plates.

Serve plated food from the right-hand side of a guest
Plates can be placed in front of the guest with the right hand and the stack of other plated food is then behind the customer's chair in the left hand. If there is an accident, then the plates held in the left hand will go onto the floor rather than over the customer. Plated foods should also be placed so that the food items are consistently in the same position for all guests.

Serve beverages from the right-hand side of a guest
Glasses are placed on the right-hand side of a cover and the service of beverages follows from this. Also, for individual drinks and for other beverages any tray is held behind the customer's seat in the server's left hand. The service of beverages such as coffee and tea also are served from the right.

Avoid leaning over customers
This is courtesy and respect for physical space. Also, no matter how clean service staff are, food smells do tend to cling to service uniforms.

Use underplates
Used (cold) for four main purposes: to improve presentation on the table; to make carrying of soup plates, bowls and other bowl shaped dishes easier; to isolate the hand from hot dishes and to allow cutlery to be carried along with the item.

Use service flats or service plates (with napkins on them to prevent items slipping)

Used for five main purposes: to improve presentation of items to be served; to make carrying of bowl shaped serving dishes easier and more secure (and avoiding the thumb of the server being inside of a service dish); to allow for more than one serving dish to be carried at one time; to isolate the hand from hot dishes and to allow service gear to be carried along with the item(s).

Hold flats, dishes and round trays on the palm of the hand

This is safer. Where the flats or dishes are hot then the service cloth can be underneath folded and laid flat onto the palm to protect the hand.

Use doilies/dish papers on underplates

Doilies, dish papers (or linen or paper napkins) on underplates are used to improve presentation, to reduce noise and to help to prevent the dish being carried from slipping on the underplate. General guide: use doilies for sweet food items and dish papers for savoury food items.

Serve cold food before hot food

When the hot food is served the service is complete and customers can enjoy the meal without waiting for additional items to be served. For the same reason accompaniments should be automatically offered and served at the same time as the food item.

Serve wine before food

Similar to above. Customers want to enjoy the wine with the meal and do not want to wait for wine service with hot food going cold.

Clear from the right-hand side of a guest

Plates can be removed from in front of the guest with the right hand and the stack of plates is then behind the customer's chair, in the waiter's left hand. If there is an accident, then the plates held in the left hand will go onto the floor rather than over the customer.

Deal with complaints or other problems quickly and discretely

Immediate attention reduces risk of problems escalating, and discretion reduces the potential for a simple problem to be become a much larger one.

Sequence banquet/function staff line-ups

Waiters serving the main guests, and the stations furthest from the service door, should be into the room first. This is courtesy and operational sense; otherwise service staff can fall over each other.

Separate the serving at table from food/drink collection and station clearing

Ensures that there is always someone in the room to attend to guests and to monitor the overall service whilst others are bringing in food and drink orders or clearing items away from the service station. This approach also allows for the training of new staff and ensures that customer contact is primarily through experienced staff.

Pass other members of staff by moving to the right

Having an establishment rule about moving to the right (or left) avoids confusion and accidents, as it ensures that all staff when meeting each other, pass or walk by each other by always moving to the right.

Hold glasses or cups at the base or by the handle

This is hygienic practice. Service staff holding glasses or cups etc. by the rim is not hygienic practice.

Avoid contact between fingers and mouth or hair

If contact between fingers and mouth or hair etc. is unavoidable then it is important, hygienically, to ensure that hands are washed before continuing with service. Also, always wash hands after using toilets.

Cover cuts and sores

Covering cuts and sores with waterproof plasters or dressings is essential hygienic practice.

Report illnesses

Any illnesses should be reported to management so that decisions can be made about fitness to work. This is for the protection of other staff as well as guests.

PART 2: WINE AND OTHER DRINKS

INTRODUCTION TO WINE

Wine is fermented grape juice, the best quality being produced mostly within the latitudes 30–50° north, and south, of the Equator. There are four main families of wine-producing vines: *Vitis vinifera* (wine bearing), which produces all the great wines, and *Vitis riparia*, *Vitis labrusca* and *Vitis rupestris*, which make less-fine wines.

Wine making has never been easy, and wine growers have had to contend with and protect their vines from all kinds of pests and diseases. The worst pest of all was the dreadful *Phylloxera vastatrix*. This aphid was brought from North America to Europe in the latter half of the nineteenth century. It attacked the vine roots and devastated most of the world's vineyards. Later on it was discovered that American rootstocks (e.g. *Vitis rupestris*) were resistant to the disease. Thus, today most vines are grafted on to American stocks.

The grape

The grape is made up of skin, stalk, pips, pulp water, sugar and acids.

The *must* (unfermented grape juice) will also have trace elements of nitrogenous compounds such as albumen, peptones, amides, ammonium salts and nitrates, as well as potassium, phosphoric acid and calcium, all of which have an influence on the eventual taste of the wine.

How wine is made

The making of wine starts with the gathering of the grapes (the vintage). The grapes are crushed to produce the *must*. Fermentation takes place, which can last from one week to three weeks, and this is the action of yeast (found on the bloom covering the outside skin of the grape) on the sugar in the *must*, converting it into ethyl alcohol and carbon dioxide gas (CO_2) through a series of complex biochemical reactions. The gas forms bubbles on the surface before escaping into the air. The yeasts continue to convert the sugar up to a maximum of 16 per cent alcohol by volume.

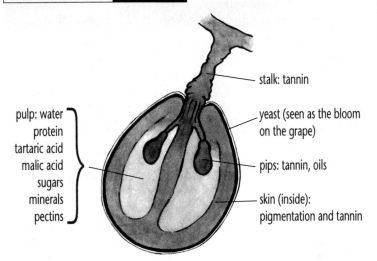

stalk: tannin

pulp: water
protein
tartaric acid
malic acid
sugars
minerals
pectins

yeast (seen as the bloom on the grape)

pips: tannin, oils

skin (inside): pigmentation and tannin

Most table wines however, have an alcoholic strength of between 10 per cent and 14 per cent.

The new wine is usually transferred to casks where it will be *racked* from time to time as it matures. The purpose of *racking* is to eliminate the *lees* (sediment or deposit) in the wine. This deposit is left behind as the wine is moved to a fresh cask and so, with each *racking*, the wine becomes clearer. Before being bottled the wine is *fined* to remove unwanted particles held in suspension. Isinglass, egg whites, gelatine and dried albumen are particularly good *fining* agents as they attract the unwanted particles and drag them down to the bottom of the cask, thus leaving behind brilliant wine, which may also be filtered before bottling. The longer the wine matures in cask the less time it needs in bottle. Great wines are matured for many years in bottle.

Factors that influence the quality of wine

Several factors influence the quality of wine. These are:

Red Wine

BLACK GRAPES

DE-STALKING
MACHINE

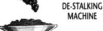

May or may
not be used

CRUSHER

Crushed grapes

FERMENTING
VESSEL

Skins are
left with juice

PRESS extracts
remaining
wine

Free-run wine
is transferred
to cask

MATURING
CASK

New wine is
racked from time
to time and may
then be fined
and/or refined

Bottled
for
maturing
or drinking

White Wine

BLACK GRAPES
or
WHITE GRAPES

DE-STALKING
MACHINE

CRUSHER
May or may
not be used

Crushed or
whole grapes

PRESS

Grape juice

FERMENTING
VESSEL

If white grapes
are used, the
skins may be left
with the juice
during fermen-
tation. If black
grapes are used
the juice is
separated before
the grape skins
impart colour

MATURING
CASK

New wine may
be racked or
left with its lees

Bottled
for
maturing
or drinking

Rosé Wine

BLACK GRAPES

DE-STALKING
MACHINE

CRUSHER

May or may
not be used

PRESS

No. 1
FERMENTING
VESSEL

Grape skins
left with the
juice until a
pink colour is
obtained from
the skins

No. 2 FERMENTING
VESSEL

The wine finishes
fermenting away
from the skins

MATURING
CASK

New wine is racked
from time to time

Bottled
for
maturing
or drinking

How wine is made

31

- Type of soil
- Climate
- Microclimate
- Aspect (site of vineyard)
- Terroir (complete growing environment)
- Grape variety
- Viticulture (the cultivation of the vine)
- Vinification (wine making)
- Luck of the year

Wine styles

Red wine

Red wine comes from black grapes that are fermented throughout with their skins and sometimes also with their stalks. As fermentation continues the alcohol generated draws colour from the inside of the skins.

Rosé wine

Rosé wine comes from black grapes without the stalks and is made in a similar way to red wine, but the juice is separated once the desired degree of pinkness has been achieved. Fermentation is completed in a separate vessel. Alternative methods are either to press the grapes so that some colour is extracted from the skins or to blend red and white wine together.

Blush wine

Blush wine is a new style of rosé wine originating in California in which the black grape skins are left to macerate for only a very short period with the *must*. The resulting wine has a blue-pink hue with copper highlights.

White wine

White wine comes from either black or white grapes. When black grapes are used, the juice is quickly moved to another vessel to begin and complete its fermentation. All grape juice is colourless initially. The juice from white grapes is usually left with the grape skins until fermentation is completed. Sweet white wines are made from sweet grapes, which have been affected by a phenomenon called *Botrytis cinerea*, also known as *pourriture noble* or noble rot. This intensifies the natural sugars of the grapes so that when fermentation is completed the wine remains sweet (also see *vin doux naturel* below).

Sparkling wine

When making sparkling wine, a sugar solution and special yeast culture are added first to dry table wine. The wine is then sealed and a secondary fermentation is allowed to take place:

- in a bottle (*méthode champenoise* or *méthode traditionnelle*)
- in a tank (*méthode cuve close*— also known as the Charmat or bulk method)
- in a bottle and then the wine is transferred under pressure to a tank or vat where it is filtered and rebottled (*méthode transuasement* transfer method)
- Sparkling wine can also be made by injecting CO_2 into the chilled vats of still wine and then bottling the wine under pressure (*méthode gazifié*), which is also sometimes called *méthode pompe bicyclette*.

Organic wines

These wines, also known as 'green' or 'environmentally friendly' wines, are made from grapes grown without the aid of artificial insecticides, pesticides or fertiliser. The wine itself will not be adulterated in any way, save for minimal amounts of the traditional preservative, sulphur dioxide, which is controlled at source.

Alcohol-free, de-alcoholised wines and low alcohol wines

- alcohol-free—maximum 0.05 per cent alcohol
- de-alcoholised—maximum 0.5 per cent alcohol
- low alcohol—maximum 1.2 per cent alcohol

These wines are made in the normal way and the alcohol is then removed either by the hot treatment, distillation (which unfortunately removes most of the flavour as well), or, more satisfactorily, by the cold filtration process, also known as reverse osmosis. This removes the alcohol by mechanically separating or filtering out the molecules of alcohol through membranes made of cellulose of acetate. The wine is repeatedly passed through the membranes in order to filter out the alcohol and water, leaving behind a syrupy wine concentrate. To this, at a later stage, water and a little *must* are added, thus preserving much of the flavour or mouthfeel of the original wine.

Vins doux naturels

These are sweet wines that have had their fermentation muted by the addition of alcohol to retain their natural sweetness. The final alcoholic strength is about 17 per cent by volume. A well-known example is Muscat de Beaumes-de-Venise.

Fortified wines

Fortified wines (known as liqueur wines in the EU), such as sherry, port and Madeira, are those that have been strengthened by the addition of alcohol, usually a grape spirit.

Aromatised wines

These are flavoured and usually fortified. Typical examples are vermouths and Commandaria.

Faults in wine

Here are the more common causes of faults in wine:

Corked wines

These are wines affected by a diseased cork caused through bacterial action or excessive bottle age. The wine tastes and smells foul. Not to be confused with cork residue in wine, which is harmless.

Maderisation or oxidation

This is caused by bad storage—too much exposure to air, often because the cork has dried out in these conditions. The colour of the wine browns or darkens and the taste very slightly resembles Madeira, hence the name. The wine tastes 'spoilt'.

Acetification

Acetification is caused when the wine is overexposed to air. The vinegar microorganism develops a film on the surface of the wine and acetic acid is produced making the wine taste sour resembling wine vinegar (*vinaigre*).

Tartrate flake

This is the crystallisation of potassium bitartrate. These crystal-like flakes, sometimes seen in white wine, may cause anxiety to some customers as they spoil the appearance of the wine which is otherwise perfect to drink. If the wine is stabilised before bottling, this condition should not occur.

Excess sulphur dioxide (SO$_2$)

Sulphur dioxide is added to wine to preserve it and keep it healthy. Once the bottle is opened the stink will disappear and, after a few minutes, the wine is perfectly drinkable.

Secondary fermentation

This happens when traces of sugar and yeast are left in the wine in bottle. It leaves the wine with an unpleasant, prickly taste that should not be confused with the *petulant, spritzig* characteristics associated with other styles of healthy and refreshing wines.

Foreign contamination

Examples include splintered or powdered glass caused by faulty bottling machinery or re-used bottles which previously held some kind of disinfectant.

Hydrogen sulphide (H$_2$S)

The wine has the characteristic smell of rotten eggs.

Sediment, lees, crust or dregs

This comprises organic matter discarded by the wine as it matures in cask or bottle. It can be removed by racking, fining or, in the case of bottled wine, by decanting.

Cloudiness

This is caused by suspended matter in the wine disguising its true colour. It may be due to extremes in storage temperatures.

SERVICE OF WINE

All wine should be properly temperatured. Approximate service temperatures for wines are:

- Champagne and sparkling wines   4.5–7°C (40–45°F)
- Sweet white wines   7–10°C (45–50°F)
- White and rosé wines   10–12.5°C (50–55°F)
- Young light red wines   12.5–15°C (55–60°F)
- Full-bodied red wines   15.5–18°C (60–65°F)

Opening techniques

In the restaurant it is very important to show the host the bottle with the label uppermost and to nominate the wine verbally to the customer so there is no confusion regarding the wine or vintage ordered.

Red wine bottles are usually placed on a coaster beside the host, whereas sparkling, white, blush and rosé bottles should be placed in a wine bucket holding ice and water up to the neck of the bottle. Trim around the top of the capsule to expose the cork. Then extract the cork carefully using a corkscrew with a wide thread so that the cork can be levered out without any crumbling. Smell the cork, which should smell of wine. Sometimes a wine may have a bit of bottle stink due to stale air being lodged between cork and wine, but this soon disappears as the wine is exposed to air.

Pour, twist and take

When pouring wine, the neck of the bottle should be over the glass, but not resting on the rim in case of an accident. Care should be taken to avoid splashing and, having finished pouring, the bottle should be twisted as it is being taken away. This will prevent drips of wine falling on the tablecloth or on someone's clothes. Any drops on the rim of the

Alsace and German

Anjou

Jura

Bordeaux

Franconia

Burgundy
and Rhône

Champagne
and sparkling

Côtes
de Provence

table
wines

Chianti

bottle should be wiped away with a clean service cloth or napkin. The host gets a small taster and decides that the wine is perfectly sound for drinking. Service proceeds on the right from the right around the table with the label clearly visible and with the host's glass being finally topped-up to the customary two-thirds full. Later, if another bottle of the same is ordered, the host should be given a fresh glass from which to taste the new wine.

Opening and serving Champagne and sparkling wines

Champagne and sparkling wines should not be shaken on their journey to the table and the wine should be well chilled. This helps control the effervescence and imparts the refreshing qualities associated with such wines.

Loosen or take off the wire muzzle. Holding the bottle at an angle of 45° in one hand and the cork in the other, twist the bottle only and, when the cork begins to move, restrain it by pushing it almost back into the neck. Soon the cork will leave the bottle quietly (never with a loud pop or bang). Should the cork prove stubborn and reluctant to leave the bottle, soak a napkin in hot water, wrap it around the neck of the bottle and movement will occur quickly.

Be extra careful when opening sparkling wines. Always keep the palm of your hand over the cork to prevent accidents to the eyes and elsewhere. Hold the bottle with your thumb in the punt and pour the wine against the inside of the glass. There should be a nice mousse but no frothing over.

Decanting

The main reasons for decanting an old red wine are (a) to separate it from the sediment, (b) to allow the wine to breathe and (c) to develop its bouquet. Fine old red wines and some ports, which have spent most of their lives maturing in bottle, throw a deposit or crust which, if allowed to enter the glass, would sully the appearance of the wine. This deposit forms as the wine ages and consists of tannins, bitartrates of calcium and magnesium and colouring matter. It makes the wine cloudy and can cause it to taste of *lees*.

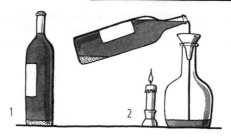

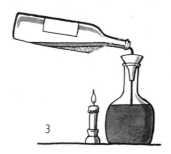

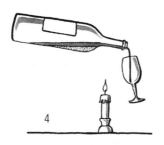

Decanting Wine

Decanting is the movement of wine from its original container to a fresh glass receptacle, leaving the grunge or sediment behind. It is best to stand the bottle upright for two days before decanting to give the sediment a chance to settle at the bottom.

1   Extract the cork carefully it may disintegrate because of long contact with alcohol, so be wary;

2   Place a light behind the shoulder of the bottle, a candle if you are decanting in front of guests, but a torch, light bulb or any light source at home or in the cellar will do;

3   Carefully pour the wine through a funnel into an absolutely clean decanter. The light will reveal the first sign of sediment entering the neck of the bottle;

4   At this stage stop pouring into the decanter but continue pouring into a glass, which should be handy. The latter wine when it settles can be used as a taster or for sauces in the kitchen.

A quick method for decanting is to place a coffee filter or perfectly clean muslin in a funnel, which should be in the neck of the decanter as the wine flows in. The vogue nowadays is also to decant younger red wines, simply because exposure to air improves the bouquet, and softens and mellows the wine. Of course, the host's permission should always be given before decanting a wine in a restaurant. Decanting also enhances the appearance of the wine, especially when presented in a fine wine decanter.

Very old red wine breaks up with too much exposure to air. It is best to stand such a bottle for a few days to allow the sediment to settle in the bottom. Then open the bottle just before the meal is served and pour the wine very carefully straight into the glass with the bottle held in the pouring position as each glass is approached. This prevents the wine slopping back to disturb the sediment. Sufficient glasses should be available to finish the bottle, thereby ensuring that the wine does not remingle with its sediment at the end of service.

Wine cradles or wine baskets are useful when taking old red wines from the cellar as they hold the bottle in the binned position, thus leaving the sediment undisturbed. If great care is taken when pouring, you can avoid disturbing the sediment by using the cradle, but the skill requires expertise and a large hand to span the cradle. It has also become fashionable to serve red wines in a wine basket. While this practice appeals to some, there is no technical argument for doing so.

Carafe wines, also known as house wines, should be pleasant to drink and may be red, white or rosé. Unlike the decanter, which is often made of cut glass and has a stopper fitted, a carafe is usually plain, of clear glass and without a stopper.

Desperate situations, desperate remedies

Wines can be chilled quickly by placing a bottle in a wine bucket containing, salt, ice and water. The salt quickly melts the ice and drastically reduces the temperature. Another way is to place the wine in the freezer for about 10 minutes. A cool red wine can be brought to room temperature by being poured into a warmed decanter or by microwaving it for about 45 seconds. However these are extreme situations and it is always best to use traditional methods of chilling or chambréing wines.

How to prevent wasting wine

Wine that is left over in a bottle, even when securely corked, becomes lifeless and unpalatable after a couple of days, so down the drain it goes. To prevent this waste, a neat piece of equipment exists called a Vacu-vin, which will reseal an opened bottle of wine, keeping the contents in perfect condition for several days. It extracts the air from the bottle and then reseals it with a special reusable stopper that preserves the natural freshness of the wine for a longer period, allowing you to drink as much as you like, when you like. There is also a sparkling wine bottle re-sealer, which is particularly useful for Champagne and other bottles of sparkling wine.

WINE TASTING

Tasting uses all the senses:

- Eyes to assess the clarity and the colour
- Smell to assess the bouquet or aroma. Taste is 80 per cent smell!
- Taste to sense the sweetness, dryness, acidity, alcohol, tannin, intensity etc.
- Touch to feel the weight, temperature etc.
- Hear to create associations with the occasion

Tasting Technique

After assessing the clarity, colour and the smell, take a small amount of the wine in the mouth together with a little air and roll it around so that it reaches the different parts of the tongue. Lean forward so that the wine is nearest the teeth and suck air in through the teeth. Doing this helps to highlight and intensify the flavour. At this stage and when the wine is spit out, the impressions made should be carefully noted otherwise confusion can occur. (Fortified wines etc. are often appraised by sight and smell without tasting, as are spirits).

The taste of a drink is detected in different parts of the mouth, but most essentially on the tongue. Sweetness is detected at the tip and centre of the tongue, acidity on the upper edges, saltiness on the sides and tip and bitterness at the back.

When tasting consider the following:

- Sweetness and dryness will be immediately obvious;
- Acidity will be recognised by its gum-drying sensation, but in correct quantities acidity provides crispness and liveliness to a drink;
- Astringency or tannin content, usually associated with red wines, will give a dry coating or furring effect especially on the teeth and gums;
- Body, which is the feel of the wine in your mouth, and flavour, the essence of the wine as a drink, will be the final arbiters as to whether you like it or not;

- Aftertaste is the finish the wine leaves on your palate, and
- Overall balance is the evaluation of all the above elements taken together.

Common aroma associations are:

Cabernet Sauvignon	Blackcurrants	Pinot Noir	strawberries, cherries, plums (depending on where grown)
Chardonnay	ripe melon, fresh pineapple		
Chenin Blanc	apples	Riesling	apricots, peaches
Gewürztraminer	tropical fruits such as lychees	Sauvignon Blanc	gooseberries
		Syrah	raspberries
Merlot	plum, damson	Zinfandel	blackberries, bramble, spice
Nebbiolo	prunes		

Other aroma associations can be as diverse as pine trees, resin, vanilla, coffee, tea, herbs, smoke, toast, leather, cloves, cinnamon, nutmeg, ginger, mint, truffles, oak, figs, lilac and jasmine.

Always make notes on what is being tasted. This helps to reinforce the learning.

MATCHING WINE AND OTHER DRINKS TO FOOD

Overall the intention is to provide food and wine that harmonise well together, each enhancing the other's performance. The combinations that prove most successful are those that please the individual. Some general guidelines are:

- Dry wines served before sweeter wines;
- White wines before red wines;
- Lighter wines before heavier wines;
- Good wines before great wines;

When considering possible food and wine partnerships, there are no

Wine tasting aide-mémoire

Wine details	Name of wine, country and area of origin, quality indication (e.g. AOC, Qmp etc.), shipper, château/estate bottled, varietal, vintage, ½ bottle, bottle, magnum, price
Clarity	Clear, bright, brilliant, gleaming, sumptuous, intense, dull, grey, subdued, hazy, cloudy, pale, faded
Colour	*White wine:* Water clear, pale yellow, yellow with green tinges, straw, gold, deep yellow, brown, maderised. *Rosé wine:* Pale pink, orange-pink, onionskin, blue-pink, copper. *Red Wine:* Purple, garnet, ruby, tawny, brick-red, mahogany
Smell (nose, aroma, bouquet)	Fruity, perfumed, full, deep, spicy, fine, rich, pleasant, nondescript, flat, corky
Taste	Bone dry, dry, medium dry, medium sweet, sweet, luscious, unctuous, thin, light, medium, full-bodied, acid, bitter, spicy, hard, soft, silky, smooth, tart, piquant
Conclusion (summing up)	Well-balanced, fine, delicate, rich robust, vigorous, fat, flabby, thick, velvety, harsh, weak, unbalanced, insipid, for laying down, just right, over the hill

It is important that you make up your own mind about the wine you are tasting. Do not be too easily influenced by the observations of others.

guidelines to which there are not exceptions: For example, although fish is usually served with white wine, some dishes, such as heavily sauced salmon, red mullet or a fish such as lamprey (which is traditionally cooked in red wine), can be successfully accompanied by a slightly chilled red Saint-Emilion, Pomerol or Mercury. It is also useful to identify the nature of the dish as being light or heavy so that wines can be chosen to match on that basis. Additionally when making recommendations it is also useful to identify the type and style of the wine the customer requires and also the extent to which the wine should be light or full.

Apéritifs

The name apéritif comes from the Latin *aperitivus* to open out (in this, case it is the gastric juices which are 'opened out' to give an appetite for the meal to come). Examples are:

■ Champagne, sherry, dry white wine, Madeira and vermouths are particularly good apéritifs, but they should not be drunk to excess, otherwise the food takes second place and is not likely to be appreciated;

■ Gin, with a variety of partners, is a popular apéritif: gin and tonic, gin and It (Italian vermouth), gin and French (French vermouth) and, of course, the Martini cocktail (gin and dry vermouth) and other cocktails. For those who dislike gin, vodka is the natural substitute;

■ Schnapps and pastis are also popular, as are the various bitters;

■ Whisky and soda, Kir, Buck's Fizz and sundry cocktails all help whet the appetite and get people in the mood for enjoying the meal;

■ A more simple approach is to serve the wine that will accompany the first course.

Some possible wine and food combinations

Hors-d'oeuvre

Sometimes combinations can be difficult because of overpowering dressings on salad items. However Fino or Manzanilla Sherry; Sancerre, Pinot Grigio, Sauvignon Blanc or Gewürztraminer can be tried. Also sometimes, depending on the dishes, the lighter reds

Soups

These do not really require a liquid accompaniment but Sherry or dry Port or Madeira could be tried. Consommés, turtle soup and lobster or crab bisque can be enhanced by adding a glass of heated Sherry or Madeira before serving

Terrines, pâtés and foie gras

Beaujolais or a light, young, red wine, white wines from Pinot Gris or Sauvignon Blanc grapes and also some sweet white wines

Omelettes and quiches
Difficult for wine but an Alsatian Riesling or Sylvaner could be tried

Farinaceous dishes (pasta and rice)
Classic Italian red wines such as Valpolicella, Chianti, Barolo, Santa Maddalena, or Lago di Caldaro

Fish
Oysters and shellfish
Dry white wines, Champagne, Chablis, Muscadet, Soave and Frascati

Smoked fish
White Rioja, Hock, white Graves, Verdicchio

Fish dishes with sauces
Fuller white wines such as Vouvray, Montrachet or Yugoslav Riesling

Shallow fried or grilled fish
Vinho Verde, Moselle, Californian Chardonnay, Australian Sémillon or Chardonnay

White meats
The type of wine to serve is dependent on whether the white meat (chicken, turkey, rabbit, veal or pork) is served hot or cold

Served hot with a sauce or savoury stuffing
Either a rosé such as Anjou, or light reds like Beaujolais, New Zealand Pinot Noir, Californian Zinfandel, Saint-Julien, Bourg and Burgundy (e.g. Passe-tout-grains) and Corbières

Served cold
Fuller white wines such as Hocks, Gran Viña Sol, Sancerre and the rosés of Provence and Tavel

Other meats
Duck and goose
Big red wines that will cut through the fat, Châteauneuf-du-Pape, Hermitage, Barolo and the Australian Cabernet Shiraz

Roast and grilled lamb
Medoc, Saint-Emilion, Pomerol and any of the Cabernet Sauvignons

Roast beef and grilled steaks
Big red Burgundies, Rioja, Barolo, Dão and wines made from the Pinot Noir grape

Meat stews
Lighter reds, Zinfandel, Côtes du Rhône, Clos du Bois, Bull's Blood, Vino Nobile di Montepulciano

Hare, venison and game
Reds with distinctive flavour, Côte Rôtie, Bourgeuil, Rioja, Chianti, Australian Shiraz, Californian Cabernet Sauvignon, Chilean Cabernet Sauvignon, and also fine red Burgundies and Bordeaux reds

Oriental foods, Peking duck, mild curry, tandoori chicken, shish kebab
Gewürztraminer, Lutomer Riesling, Vinho Verde, Mateus Rosé or Anjou Rosé. Also beers

Cheese

The wine from the main course is often followed through to the cheese course although it is also worth considering the type of cheese being served

Light, cream cheeses
Full bodied whites, rosés and light reds

Strong, pungent (even smelly) and blue-veined varieties
Big reds of Bordeaux and Burgundy, or tawny, vintage or vintage-style Ports and also the luscious sweet whites

Sweets and puddings

Champagne works well with sweets and puddings. Others to try are the luscious Muscats (de Beaumes-de-Venise, de Setúbal, de Frontignan, Samos), Sainte-Croix-du-Mont, Sauternes, Banyuls, Monbazillac, Tokay, wines made from late-gathered individual grapes in Germany and also the Orange Muscats and speciality drinks such as Vin de Frais (fermentation of fresh strawberries) both of which can go well with chocolate

Dessert (fresh fruit and nuts)

Sweet fortified wines, Sherry, Port, Madeira, Málaga, Marsala, Commandaria, Yalumba Galway Pipe and Seppelt's Para.

Coffee

Cognac and other brandies such as Armagnac, Asbach, Marc, Metaxa, Grappa, Oude Meester, Fundador, Peristiani V031

Good aged malt whiskies

Calvados, sundry liqueurs and Ports

WINE GROWING COUNTRIES

Algeria

Produces red or rosé wines in three centres: Alger, Oran and Constantine. The reds made from the Carignan, Cinsault and Alicante–Bouschet grapes. The rosés are made from the Cinsault and Grenache, and the little white that is made comes from Ugni Blanc and Clairette de Provence grapes.

Argentina

All manner of wines are produced and in huge quantities. Mendoza is the biggest and best region. Other good locations are San Juan, Río Negro, La Rioja and Juyjuy, part of Salta and Catamarca. Cabernet Sauvignon, Malbec, Merlot, Pinot Noir, Tempranillo and Syrah are the red wine grapes and the Riesling, Sauvignon Blanc and Pinot Blanc are used to make white wine. There are also sparkling wines, including one marketed as Champania 'M. Chandon'.

Australia

Produces excellent, good-value wines in a wide range of styles, sometimes blending two or more grape varieties to great advantage. The Chardonnay, Gerwürztraminer, Rhine Riesling, Sauvignon Blanc and Sémillon are the main white grapes, with the brown Muscat (Frontignac) for dessert wine. Red wines are made from the Cabernet Sauvignon, Pinot Noir, Hermitage, Shiraz and Malbec grapes.

Labels are informative, stating the grape or combination of grapes used. Sometimes they can be tricky, for example 'C S Malbec' on a label would indicate a blend, in descending proportions, of three red grapes Cabernet Sauvignon, Shiraz and Malbec. Generally, however, the labels are easy to understand, as long as they do not give too much technical information such as the baumé number (sugar level of the grape when picked), age in cask and date of bottling. Words like 'Private Bin', 'Reserve Bin' and 'Bin Number' may indicate that the wine comes from a single vineyard and is of superior quality.

The principal areas are New South Wales, not far from Sydney; in Victoria near Melbourne; in the Barossa Valley, Clare Valley, Coonawarra, along the banks of the Murray River and around Adelaide, South Australia; in Queensland near Brisbane; in Western Australia, in the Swan Valley near Perth; and in Tasmania near Hobart. Sparkling wines are made by the *méthode traditionnelle*. Australian sherry-style and port-style fortified wines are also produced. Wines are marketed under the names of producers, for example: Angas, Hill Smith, Jacob's Creek, Lindeman's, Penfolds, Rosemont, Rothbury and Yalumba.

Austria

About three-quarters of Austrian wine is white, made mostly from the native grape Grüner Veltliner, with contributions also from the Rhine Riesling, Welschriesling, Weissburgunder (Pinot Blanc), Gewürztraminer, Müller–Thurgau and Muskat-Ottonel. Red wines when made, come from the Blauer Spätburgunder (Pinot Noir), Blaufränkisch, Portugieser and Saint Laurent grapes. The most popular white wine in Austria is Gumpoldskirchner made in a village near Baden, south of Vienna from special grapes not mentioned above. They are Rotipflier and Spätrot, blended in equal proportions. Further south of Vienna the red, Vöslauer, is made in the village of Bad Vöslau. Vineyards to the west of Vienna, especially in the Wachau district, produce fine white such as Dürnsteiner Katzensprung, Dürnsteiner Flohaxen, Lóiben Kaiser wein, Riede Lóibenberg, Kremser Kögl and Kremser Wachtberg.

Burgenland in the eastern part of Austria gets lots of sunshine and has ideal conditions for producing overripe grapes, which in extreme ripeness are known as *ausbruch*. A delicious example of this is the wine from

Neusiedler See, called 'Rust'. Other wines are the white styles Neuberger, Mörbischer, St Georgener Welschriesling and the light and fruity red Blaufränkischer. In Steiermark, in the southern corner of Austria, they make a blush-style wine called Schilcher, which results from very brief maceration of the grape skins. In West Steiermark the speciality is the onion-skin-coloured rosé called Zwiebelschilcher.

Bolivia

Some light table wines are produced around La Paz and Sucre. Most wine is for home consumption or is distilled into local Pisco brandy.

Bosnia–Herzegovina

Produces two well-known dry varietal wines. Zilavka is a pungent dry white wine that comes from vineyards around the city of Mostar, and there is a mild-flavoured red wine called Blatina.

Brazil

Industry is dominated by a number of large companies, many of which are cooperatives. Wines are generally blended and sold under proprietary names. *Labrusca* varieties are grown but also increasing quantities of *vinifera* varieties. Grapes for red wine are Cabernet Sauvignon, Cabernet Franc, Merlot and Barbera, and Trebbiano, Chardonnay and Sémillion for whites.

Bulgaria

One of the world's largest producers and exporters of very good and reasonably priced wines. They are matured in oak cask; whites for up to 18 months and the reds for three years. Whites to look out for are Dimiat, Riesling, Chardonnay, Sauvignon Blanc and Misket, and the reds Gamza, Mavrud, Melnic and Cabernet Sauvignon all are generous, soft and rounded in flavour.

Canada

Ontario is by far the biggest and most important wine region. Much of the wine comes from the *Vitis labrusca* family (Concorde, Catawba, Delaware, Niagara and President). In more recent times the *Vitis vinifera* varietals have been cultivated, such as Aligoté, Chardonnay,

Gewürztraminer and the Johannisberg Riesling for whites and the Pinot Noir and Gamay for reds. Besides the red and white table wines, dessert-style wines, including Eiswein, and a substantial amount of sparkling wines are made.

Chile

Chile's red wines, especially the Cabernet Sauvignons, are world class. Look out for this style from Concha y Toro, Cousino Macul, Miguel Torres and Santa Rita. They are full, rich and velvet smooth, certain to please both palate and pocket. The best Chilean wines come from the Maipo and Aconcagua valleys. Reds are also produced either as blenders, or in their own right, from Cabernet Franc, Malbec, Merlot and Pinot Noir grapes. Torres also produces a good rosé from the Cabernet Sauvignon grape and a refreshing sparkling white made by the *méthode traditionnelle*. The still whites have not, as yet, reached the same high standards as the reds but again Torres Sauvignon Blanc has good balance and elegance. The Chardonnay and Sémillon grapes are also used to produce sound whites.

China

China makes some rice 'wine' and white wines called Dynasty, Heavenly Palace and Great Wall. A sweet wine called Meikuishanputaochu is also made, as is a red wine called Cabernet d'Est. Climatic conditions are against quality.

Croatia

Produces mostly red wine, with the black Plavac Mali grape widely cultivated, One of the best wines is the full-bodied Dingac made from semi-dried grapes. Other good reds are Postup, Faros, Bolski Plavaè and Motovunski Teran. Inland there is a light, straw coloured wine called Kutjevacka Grasevina. Near the Hungarian border in Kontinentalna Hrvatska the Lash Riesling grape makes an abundance of semi-sweet white wines. GRK is a sherry-style wine made in the island of Korčula.

Cyprus

Produces a selection of wines running from dry, medium and the more popular sweet sherry-style wines, to the renowned dessert wine,

Commandaria. Although the sherry-type wines are the more popular, Commandaria, reckoned to be the oldest known wine in the world, has more distinction (wine flavoured with cloves, resin, scented wood, and fortified with local brandy to produce a honey-sweet, amber-red wine).

The island also produces light whites: Amathus, Arsinoe, Palomino; medium whites: Aphrodite, Bellapais (white and rosé semi-sparkling) and Thisbe; sweet whites: Hirondelle, St Hilarion and St Panteleimon; rosé wine: including Coeur de Lion, Amorosa and Kokkineli, a deep rosé wine; red wine: the mellow Kykko, Olympus and Salamis, the dry and flavoursome Agravani and the full-bodied and fragrant Mames, Kolossi and Othello. Sparkling wines are also produced.

Czech Republic and Slovakia

The main producing areas are in the regions of Bohemina and Moravia and the state of Slovakia. Most of the wine is white—still and sparkling—and made from Reinriesling, Vlässkyrizling, Grüner Veltliner, Sylvana, Müller–Thurgau, Gewürztraminer and Rulandské grapes. Red wines are made from the Limberger and Spätburgunder (Pinot Noir) grapes. A golden sweet, Tokay-style wine is also made using the Furmint, Härslevelü and Muscat grapes.

Egypt

Although wine was made in Egypt in ancient times, it was the 20th century that saw a resurgence. Native grapes, Fayumi and Rumi, as well as Chardonnay, Chasselas, Pinot Noir, Muscat Hamburg, Gamay and Pinot Noir are cultivated. Wines are sold under names such as Reine Cléopâtre and Cru des Ptolemées for whites and the red Omar Khyyam.

England

'English' wines are made from grapes grown in England alone. Wines labelled 'British' are made from imported unfermented grape juice (*must*) and cannot be called 'English' wines. The vine was first introduced into Britain by the Romans and was cultivated from then on. When Eleanor of Aquitaine married Henry II in 1152, part of her dowry was the lands of Bordeaux, which England owned thereafter for some 300 years. The red wine of Bordeaux was markedly superior to the wines of England and this fact, together with the dissolution of the monasteries in the 1530s, resulted in many vineyards falling into disuse. It was not until the middle of the 20th Century that the English wine industry resurfaced physically and commercially.

Today in England and Wales there are more than 300 vineyards occupying over 405 hectares (1,000 acres), producing mainly white wines from Germanic vine strains. These strains are especially suited to cold, northerly vineyards, with the extreme limit of cultivation being a rough line across the country from The Wash. Grapes include: Müller-Thurgau, Schönburger, Ortega, Reichensteiner, Huxelrebe, Bacchus, Gütenborner, Seyve Villard, Modo Muscat, Riesling and Sylvaner, and a French hybrid, Seyval Blanc. There are also red and rosé wines made from Pinot Noir, Zweigeltrebe and Gamay grapes. Look out for the EVA quality seal, which is awarded annually by the English Viticultural Association to wines that are submitted for official testing.

France

The glorious wine gardens of France produce a diversity of wine styles, generally of noble quality. Besides the excellent natural aspects of soil and climate, quality is controlled at all stages of production. The levels of quality are:

- **Vins de table:** this is ordinary table wine in the cheapest price range. It is not recognized under quality control standards.

- **Vins de pays:** the lowest official category recognized. Wines of medium quality and price, made from certain grapes grown within a defined area. The area must be printed on the label. A minimum alcohol content is specified.

- **Vins délimité de qualité supérieure (VDQS):** A quality wine just below appellation controlled standard. Area of production, grape varieties, minimum alcohol content, cultivation and vinification methods are specified.

- **Appellation d'origine contrôlée (AC or AOC):** Quality wine from approved areas. Grape varieties and proportions, pruning and cultivation method, maximum yield per hectare, vinification and minimum alcohol content are specified.

Alsace

Alsace wines are mainly white after the style of German Rhine wines and are marketed in tall green *flûte d'Alsace* bottles under grape rather than place names. Alsace Riesling is probably the most popular wine but other grapes used are Gewürztraminer, Pinot Gris (Tokay), Pinot Blanc (Klevner), Muscat and Sylvaner. The Pinot Noir is used to make a little red and a rosé known as Clairet d'Alsace or Schillerwein. There is also a white wine, Alsace Edelzwicker, made from a blend of noble grapes such as Riesling, Sylvaner, etc. The sparkling Crémant d'Alsace is made mostly from a combination of Riesling and Pinot grapes. Alsace wines have variety in style and flavour and are reliably well made. The region is also famous for its Alcool Blanc, notably Eau-de-Vie de Poire William.

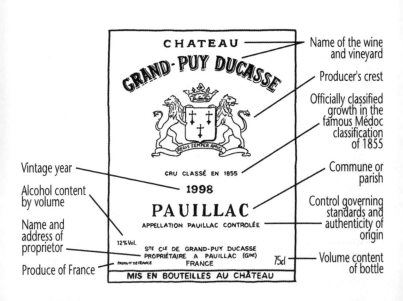

Name of the wine and vineyard

Producer's crest

Officially classified growth in the famous Médoc classification of 1855

Commune or parish

Control governing standards and authenticity of origin

Volume content of bottle

Vintage year

Alcohol content by volume

Name and address of proprietor

Produce of France

CHATEAU
GRAND-PUY DUCASSE
REGIS SEMPER AMICE
CRU CLASSÉ EN 1855
1998
PAUILLAC
APPELLATION PAUILLAC CONTROLÉE
12% Vol.
STE CIE DE GRAND-PUY DUCASSE
PROPRIÉTAIRE A PAUILLAC (GDE)
PRODUIT DE FRANCE
FRANCE
75cl
MIS EN BOUTEILLES AU CHÂTEAU

Some French wine terms

Château/domaine	estate
Crémant	less sparkling than mousseux
Cru	(growth) used to describe a single vineyard; Grand cru and premier grand cru indicate higher and highest quality vineyards
Cuve close	sparkling wine made in bulk inside a sealed vat
Cuvée	blend or contents of a vat of wine
Méthode Champenoise	Champagne method used in making some sparkling wines; now known as *méthode traditionnelle*
Millésime	vintage date
Mis en bouteille a la propriété par	bottled at the property or estate for somebody else, usually a wine dealer
Mis en bouteille au château/domaine	bottled at the estate
Mis en bouteille dans nos caves/chais	bottled in our cellars, usually by a large wine company: not estate bottled
Moelleux	sweetish and smooth
Mousseux	sparkling
Négociant	wine handler who buys bulk wine from growers and sells it under own label
Pétillant	lightly sparkling
Propriétaire, Récoltant	owner, grower
Récolte	harvested—followed by the vintage year
Sec	dry (demi-sec: medium dry and doux: sweet)
Sur lie	wine left to mature on its lees (sediment) before being bottled
Vendange tardive	late harvested grapes, which produce sweeter wine
Vin Primeur	(Vin de l'année, Vin nouveau) wine made to be drunk within a year

Bordeaux

Some 70 per cent of the total production of wine in Bordeaux is AOC quality, of which two-thirds are red and one-third white. The red wines are made from the Cabernet Sauvignon, Cabernet Franc, Merlot, Malbec and Petit Verdot grapes and the whites from the Sémillon, Sauvignon Blanc and Muscadelle grapes. The main wine growing areas are: Médoc, Saint Emilion, Pomerol, Fronsac, Côtes de Castellion and Côtes de Francs, Entre-Deux-Mers, Graves, Cérons, Sauternes, and Bourg and Blaye.

Médoc
The most famous area in the world for the production of quality, long-lasting red wines. The area is so renowned for fine wines that in 1855, 61 of the better wines were classified into five divisions known as crus, or growths, and that classification, with just a few exceptions, holds good to this day. Included within the Médoc boundaries are the principal areas of Listrac, Margaux, Moulis, Pauillac, Saint-Estèphe and Saint-Julian.

Saint Emilion
Famous red wine district making red wines, predominantly from the Merlot grape, blended with lesser amounts of Cabernet Sauvignon and Cabernet Franc. The wines are full and rounded with Château Ausone and Château Cheval Blanc being fine examples. The top classification names in descending order are: Première Grand Cru Classe, Grand Cru Classe and Grand Cru. The Saint-Emilion satellites are areas adjoining Saint-Emilion, which can also add the appellation to their name. These are: Montagne Saint-Emilion, Lussac Saint-Emilion, St-Georges Saint-Emilion, Puisseguin Saint-Emilion.

Pomerol
Neighbouring district, to the west of Saint-Emilion, produces rich meaty but smooth reds; Château Pétrus is the best known.

Fronsac and Cannon-Fronsac
Red wine area situated west of Libourne. Similar to Pomerol the dominant grape is Merlot.

Côtes de Castellion and Côtes de Francs
These two relatively new appellations situated to the east of Saint-Emilion and its surrounding satellites, produce red and white (dry and sweet) wines.

Entre-Deux-Mers

A stretch of land between the two rivers Garonne and Dordogne produces decent reds plus dry and sweet white wines. AOC is at present limited to the dry white wines; the others may be sold as Bordeaux or Bordeaux Supérieure.

Graves

Both red and white wines are made, although it is the reds that have the better reputation, especially the outstanding Château Haut-Brion, which was nominated as a premier cru (first growth) wine in the famous 1855 classification of the Médoc.

Cérons

This area is on the borders of Graves, producing white fragrant wines, which vary in style from dry to extremely sweet.

Sauternes

Produces the most remarkable naturally sweet, golden wine due to the phenomenon called *Botrytis cinerea,* also known as *pourriture noble* or noble rot. The resulting wine, luscious with creaminess and intense sweetness, has a vigour about it that stands it apart from other sweet wines. This quality is best exemplified by the famous Château d'Yquem. Also within the limitations of the Sauternes boundaries are the regions of Barsac, Bommes, Fargues and Preignac, all producing very good sweet wines.

Bourg and Blaye

These two areas produce white and red wines, but they are probably best known for, their bright, full-bodied robust reds of Cru Bourgeois quality.

Burgundy

The vineyards of Burgundy stretch from Chablis in the far north to Lyon in the south, producing, in good years, white and red wines of excellence. However, in some years the grapes in the more northerly limitations do not ripen properly and wine producers take over from nature to add sugar to the *must* to bring the alcohol content up to that of a similar wine produced in a good year. This doctoring of the wine is legal and is known as chaptalisation after Dr Chaptal (1756–1832) who first introduced the practice. Chaptalised wines cannot be sold as vintage wines, they do not even bear that stamp of class and are often sold as second-name wines or co-operative wines. This means that a vintage on a Burgundy label really means something.

Of all the wine produced, five-sixths is red and only one-sixth white. The great reds are made from the classic Pinot Noir grape and others from the Gamey or Passe-tout-grains (a mixture of one-third Pinot Noir and two-thirds Gamay). The excellent whites are produced from Chardonnay grapes and the rest mainly from the Aligoté.

Multi-ownership of original vineyards is a tradition with many of the finest wines being domaine bottled by the grower and sold under the vineyard or *commune* (parish) label. Much is also sold to *négociants* who prepare a blend of several wines, thereby averaging the quality as well as the price.

Burgundy is divided into six regions: Chablis, Côte de Nuits, Côte de Beaune, Côte Chalonnaise, Côte Mâconnaise and Beaujolais.

Chablis
The flinty dry white wines coming from this district have attained the greatest possible distinction, being generally regarded as the best accompaniment to shellfish and light delicate foods. Going from basic to brilliant, the wines are classified as Petit Chablis, Chablis, Chablis Premier Cru and Chablis Grand Cru. The latter has seven vineyards of the highest calibre: Vaudésir, Grenouilles, Blanchots, Les Preuses, Les Clos, Les Bougros and Valmur

Côte de Nuits
Red wine district of great renown producing full-bodied meaty wines, which develop gradually into silky smooth wines of exceptional class. Some examples of the famous wines are: Gevrey-Chambertin, Morey Saint-Denis, Chambolle, Musigny, Vougeot, Flagey-Echézeaux, Vosne Romanée and Nuits-Saint-George.

Côte de Beaune
District famous for fine, supple reds, which age in a reasonably short time. The reds include: Pernand-Vergelesses, Aloxe Corton, Savigny-les-

Beaune, Beaune, Pommard, Volnay, Santenay and Chassagne-Montrachet. Côte de Beaune whites are celebrated for their superb style and quality, the finest being produced in the Montrachet and neighbouring Meursault vineyards. However, there are also other fine wines from Côte de Beaune, for example Corton-Charlemagne (Aloxe Corton).

Côte de Beaune can be a combination wine from the Beaune area. Côte de Beaune Villages comes from one or more villages that have a right to the appellation.

Beaune is also known for its Hospices de Beaune, a fifteenth-century almshouse that looks after pensioners and the poor. The hospital was founded in 1443 by the then Chancellor Nicolas Rolin who endowed the premises with vineyards and encouraged others to be benefactors in like manner. The sale of wines from these vineyards supports the Hospices.

The Côte de Nuits and Côte de Beaune are together popularly known as the Côte d'Or (Golden Hillsides), not only because of the beautiful vista of their gold-coloured vine yards in the autumn but also because of the wealth that the wines have generated.

Côte Chalonnaise
Produces lighter red wines that mature quickly. Mercurey, Rully and Givry are the best examples while Montagny, made exclusively from Chardonnay grapes, and Bouzeron are the best of the white wines made. Also produced is a sparkling wine sold as Crément de Bourgogne or Borgogne Mousseux. The main producing villages are Bouzeron, Rully, Givry, Mercury and Montagne.

Côte Mâconnaise
Prolific producer of light, red, fruity and pleasant wines. They are usually sold as Mâcon Rouge or Mâcon Supérieur and the latter must have an alcohol content of 11 per cent. The best well-known Mâconnais wine is the white Pouilly Fuissé made from Chardonnay grapes in the communes of Fuissé, Salutre, Vergisson and Chaintré. Adjoining communes, Pouilly-Vinzelles and Pouilly Loché, also produce these typically fine fresh and vigorous wines while the appellation Mâcon-Villages (Blanc) has sound

whites such as Mâcon Lugny, Mâcon Prissé and Mâcon Clessé. Saint Véran, made in vineyards that overlap Mâcon and Beaujolais, is similar in style.

Beaujolais

Although some white wine is made in Beaujolais, it is the light, fruity aromatic reds that give the area fame and fortune. Genuine Beaujolais is made in huge quantities from Gamay grapes and ranges in quality from basic Beaujolais, Beaujolais Supérieur to Beaujolais Villages (a blend of wine from two villages or more). Most wines are sold under the parish name of origin (Beaujolais Cru): Saint-Amour, Juliénas, Chénas, Chiroubles, Morgon, Moulin-à-Vent, Brouilly, Côte de Brouilly, Fleurie and Régnié

Beaujolais Nouveau (Beaujolais Primeur) accounts for half the Beaujolais sales. This light but pleasant wine is made by a method called *macération carbonique*. It is a soft, fragrant, fruity wine that is ready for drinking once bottled. It is released for sale on the third Thursday in November and is best drunk between then and Christmas. Beaujolais de l'Année is somewhat different being offered for sale within a year of its vintage.

Champagne

Champagne is a protected name and is regarded as the greatest of all sparkling wines. The vineyards are located in north-east France in three main demarcated areas: Montague de Reims, Vallée de la Marne and Côte des Blancs (the white hillsides near Epernay which are planted with the white Chardonnay grape, hence the name). The two areas are Côte de Sézanne to the south of Champagne, and The Aube which is most southerly.

Besides Chardonnay, which gives an attractive crispness, delicacy and finesse to Champagne, two black grapes are used: the Pinot Noir and the Pinot Meunier. These give body and balance to the wine. When the wine is made solely from the Chardonnay grape it is known as Blanc de Blancs (white of whites). The resulting wine is very light, refreshing and delicate. If made only from black grapes it is called Blanc de Noirs and results in a much fuller, rounded, heavier Champagne. The great majority of

Champagne is made from a combination of all three grapes, which provides a beautiful unique balance.

In addition to the sparkling champagne, which is made by the Champagne method (*méthod champenoise*), the region also produces small quantities of still white wine Coteaux champenoise, a red wine Bouzy rouge and a rosé wine Rosé des Riceys.

Terms on champagne bottles, indicating from the very dry to the lusciously sweet are: Ultra brut, Brut de Brut, Brut absolut, Dosage zero, Nature, Brut, Extra sec, Sec, Demi-sec, Demi-doux and Doux

Champagne bottle names and sizes

Quarter-bottle
Half-bottle
Bottle
Magnum—2 bottles
Jeroboam—double magnum—4 bottles
Rehoboam—6 bottles
Methuselah (methusalem)—8 bottles
Salmanazar—12 bottles
Balthazar—16 bottles
Nebuchadnezzar—20 bottles

Styles of Champagne

- *Luxury Cuvée:* Made by some firms in a really outstanding year and kept aside and nurtured through every stage of its development. These include: Dom Pérignon, Tattinger Comtes de Champagne, Dom Ruinart, Pol Roger Winston Churchill and Roderer Cristal

- *Vintage Champagne:* Wine from a single good year (although this may include up to 20 per cent of a wine from another specific year to assist the blend).

- *Non-vintage Champagne:* Blend of wines from different years.

- *Pink Champagne:* Available as vintage or non-vintage and made by leaving the grape skins with the must until the juice becomes pink in colour. It is also made by blending together red and white wines.

- *Grandes Marques Champagnes:* Certain houses hold this distinction because they consistently produce excellent high-quality Champagne. These include: Ayala, Bollinger, Canard Duchêne, Veuve Clicquot Ponsardin, G H Mumm, Heidsieck Monopole, Krug, Lanson, Louis Roederer, Moet et Chandon, Perrier Jouet, Piper Heidsieck, Pol Roger, Pommery & Greno, Ruinart and Tattinger

- *Buyer's Own Brand (BOB):* Some firms will make a Champagne for a restaurant or a chain of restaurants that will be sold under the buyer's own label.

- *Recently Disgorged (Recemment Degorgé) (RD):* Special wines left to mature with their sediment in bottle for many years to produce a fine, full-flavoured, and balanced wine. They are usually released for sale after about 8 to 10 years, but can remain healthy for much longer.

Corsica

Corsica, the largest of France's islands produces good red and white table wine, some of which has the Vin de Corse Appellation Contrôlée distinction; The red Patrimonio is well acclaimed, as is the white Vin de Corse Porto-Vecchio. A feature of Corsican wine is its high alcohol content. Cap Corse is a rusty red, medium sweet, wine-based apéritif that is popular on the island.

Jura

In the districts of Arbois, Côtes du Jura and L'Etoile red, white and rosé (*vinsgris*) wines are made. Many are sold under the Arbois appelation. Côtes du Jura Mousseux is the finest of the sparkling wine appellations. Some unique wines are also made in the Jura such as Vin Jaune (yellow wine), Vin de Paille (straw wine) and Macvin. Vin Jaune is made from Sauvignon grapes. It is a pale, golden wine after the style of fino sherry but with an austere dryness and hazelnut flavour, and an alcoholic strength of 15 per cent. A good example, Château Chalon, is traditionally sold in a dumpy bottle called a clavelin. Vini de Paille is a dessert wine gets its name from the fact that the grapes are laid out on straw (*paille*) to dry and partially shrink them before pressing. Sometimes the grapes are hung from rafters during the winter to concentrate the juice. The finished wine has a flavour of quinces. Macvin is an apéritif wine, which is fairly similar to white port, and is fortified with local *eau-de-vie-de-marc* and flavoured with ingredients such as coriander and cinnamon. It is best served chilled and is also nice with ice.

Savoie

Savoie is situated between Lyon and Geneva. The area is noted for its still and sparkling white wine. Best whites are Crépy, Apremont, Seyssel, Roussette de Savoie and the sparkling wine Royal Seyssel made by Varichon and Clerc. The reds, often made from the Gamay and Pinot Noir grapes, are best exemplified by the Cruët and Motmélian styles.

Loire

Loire valley wines, be they produced by a co-operative or domaine bottled from a single vineyard, can be red, white, rosé and sparkling wines. The reds and better rosés are made from the Cabernet Franc grape and the whites from Sauvignon Blanc, Chenin Blanc, Muscadet and Chasselas grapes. Loire red wines are also very pleasant slightly chilled.

The Loire can be divided into four main wine-growing districts: Central Loire (around Sancerre, Pouilly Fumé, Pouilly-sur-Loire, Quincy and Reuilly), Touraine (incorporating Tours, Bougueil, Chinon and Blois), Anjou (including Angers and Saumur) and the Pays Nantais near the Atlantic coast. The best dry whites are Muscadet, Sancerre and Pouilly Blanc Fumé.

Muscadet is made from the Muscadet (Melon de Bourgogne) grape around the city of Nantes. This is a fresh dry wine with an attractive acidity. It is a popular apéritif, and goes extremely well with shellfish. The most popular style is Muscadet sur lie. The wine is left to mature in cask on its lees before bottling, which imparts freshness, depth of flavour and an intense bouquet.

Sancerre is a delightful, dry, smoky white wine. It is produced in the Cher Department in Central Loire and can be drunk young, but it improves with bottle age. Some red Sancerre from the Pinot Noir grape is also made.

Pouilly Blanc Fumé is a wine quite similar to Sancerre, but with a little more brightness and elegance. It gets its Fumé appendage not only because of its gun flint flavour, but also because of the smoky, blue, dust haze reflected by the ripe grapes over the vineyards around Pouilly-sur-Loire in the cooler autumn air.

Other Loire wines include the medium dry white wines Vouvray and Saumur. Vouvray, from near Tours in Touraine, is especially popular because of its versatility and genuine and agreeable nature. Saumur as a still wine is more difficult to obtain outside France. However, it is well marketed as a traditional method sparkling wine, as Vouvray sometimes is. It is produced in the district around Saumur, in the Anjou region of the Loire. Quarts de Chaume and Bonnezeaux are two of the better sweet white wines from the Coteaux du Layon area in Anjou. Made in the style of Sauternes, they improve as they mature. The rosé wines of Anjou are very popular and those sold as Cabernet d'Anjou are of superior quality. Of the reds, Chinon, Bourgueil, Saint-Nicolas-de-Bourgueil and Saumur Champigny are bright and fruity with a good depth of flavour.

The Midi

Languedoc and Roussillon are collectively popularly known as the belly of France, because it makes huge amounts of inexpensive table wines. It is estimated that up to 40 per cent of the total wine production of France is made here. While some of the wine is used as a base in the production of vermouth, the best quality (mostly red) is sold as Coteaux de Languedoc, Roussillon, Corbières, Fitou, Minervois and Costières du Gard.

The area is also famous for *vins doux naturels*. Made mostly from the Muscat grape and sometimes from the Grenache, the fermentation is stopped and the sweetness retained by adding alcohol to the fermenting must. The finished wines have an alcohol content of 17 per cent. The best examples include Grand Roussillon, Muscat de Frontignan, Muscat de Rivesaltes and the red Banyuls.

Blanquette de Limoux, a dry sparkling wine, is also made by the *méthod traditionnelle*. Seriously considered as the best sparkling wine outside Champagne, it has elegance and fragrance and is at its most refreshing when drunk young.

Some of the best dry white table wines are Clairette du Languedoc,

Clairette de Bellegarde from Gard, and Picpoul de Pinet from Hérault. Around Montpellier, great quantities of red, white and rosé wines, known as Vins Sables du Golfe du Lion, are produced. The vines are mostly cultivated in sand dunes and in the sandy marshes close to the Camargue. The area is especially noted for the largest single vineyard in France—Domaines des Salins du Midi—whose wines are marketed under the brand name Listel. Of particular interest is Listel Gris de Gris, a blush wine, made from free-run juice of the Grenache and Cinsault grapes.

Provence

Provence wines are generally sold in unusually shaped bottles with distinctive, almost lavish, labels. These wines in the South of France go wonderfully well with the foods and the atmosphere of the Mediterranean. Red, white and rosé wines are produced almost everywhere. The red and rosés are from the Cinsault, Cabernet Sauvignon, Grenache and Mourvèdre grapes and, the whites from the Ugni Blanc, Clairette and Macabéo, Marsanne, Rolle, and Sauvignon Blanc.

The main wine-growing regions of Provence are around Bandol, Bellet, Cassis, Palette and Côtes de Provence. Bandol produces red, white and rosé wines. The reds age well, whereas the rosés are ready for drinking within a few months. The whites, though scarce, are dry and spicy. Bellet produces red, white and rosé wines which are mostly drunk locally in the restaurants and cafés in and around Nice. Cassis also produces red, white and rosé wines are produced, with the white being predominant in quality and availability. Palette, an area near Aix-en-Provence, makes small quantities of good red wines and decent white and rosé wines. Many Provence wines are also sold under the *Côtes de Provence* label as well as under Aix-en-provence. The rosés seem to be regarded as the best.

Rhône

Vineyards of the Rhône stretch from Lyon to Avignon producing red, white and rosé wines of class. The reds are the real heavyweights: big, masculine wines, strong in alcohol and flavour. They are usually made from the Syrah grape or from a combination of Grenache, Cinsault, Carignan, Mourvèdre and others. In fact there are 13 varieties that are permitted to be used in the making of the famous Châteauneuf-du-Pape.

The outstanding reds, besides the spicy Châteauneuf, are Côte Rôtie, Hermitage, Crozes-Hermitage, Saint-Josèph, Cornas, Gigondas, Lirac, Côtes du Rhône Villages and Côtes du Ventoux.

The best whites are Château Grillet and Condrieu made from the Viognier grape. Other white grape varieties are Rousanne, Marsanne, Clairette and Ugni Blanc. Tavel is France's best rosé wine and is made predominantly from the Grenache grape. Saint-Peray is a clean, lively, sparkling wine made by the classical method, as is the better-known Clairette de Die, which can also be demi-sec or doux. The great *vin doux naturel* is Muscat de Beaumes-de-Venise which is fortified with grape brandy during fermentation to preserve its sweetness,

South West France

The main wine-producing regions in South West France are Bergerac, Cahors, Gaillac, Jurançon, Irouléguy and Madiran. Bergerac vineyards are located on both banks of the Dordogne, where the Dordogne Valley begins. The wines are red, white and rosé, but the outstanding wine of the region is the deep golden, luscious, creamy rich Monbazillac made, like Sauternes, from grapes affected by the *Botrytis cinerea* fungus. Next best are the dry reds Bergerac, Côte de Bergerac and Pécharmant. Cahors, a town on the River Lot, is famous for its dark red wines made from Malbec or Cot grapes. In youth the wines are exceptionally robust, but usually they are allowed to, age for years in cask to provide the finesse, which has made them so popular in France. The aged wines are very good, but very expensive. Gaillac is best known for its white wine made from Mauzac grapes. Some of the wine is perlé (slightly sparkling). The rosé and red wines are usually made from Gamay grapes and are mostly drunk locally. Jurançon wine growers, on the foothills of the Pyrenees, to the south and west of Pau, make mainly red and dry white wines nowadays. Some of the traditional sweet white wine called Jurançon Moelleux is still around, but it is expensive. Irouléguy produces red, white and rosé wines on the western side of the Atlantic Pyrenees on the Spanish border and some of the best reds are now available in Britain. Madiran produces mostly red wines made almost exclusively from local Tannat grapes. This deep-coloured, distinctive wine is a great favourite in the Pyrenees.

Germany

German wines are easy to drink, can be drunk on their own as a conversation wine *(Unterhaltungswein)* or with a wide variety of foods. Their fruity flavour, low alcohol, attractive balance of acid and sugar and reasonable price have particular appeal to new wine drinkers.

The majority of German wines are white and can be *trocken* (dry), *halb trocken* (less dry). Others are, sparkling white wine (known as *Sekt*), rosé wine *(Weissherbst)* made from black grapes only, *Rotling* wine from a combination of white and black grapes resulting in such specialities as *Rotgold* in Baden and *Schillerwein* (shimmering wine) in Württemberg, and red wine. Although German wines are often sold under a proprietary or brand label, many are identified by their region, district or vineyard and by the degree of grape ripeness at harvest time.

Up to 50 different species of grapes are grown in German vineyards, many of them new or experimental. The principal ones used are Riesling, Silvaner, and Müller-Thurgau (Riesling and Silvaner cross). The grape variety does not have to appear on a label but, when it does, there is a guarantee that at least 85 per cent of the wine has been produced from the indicated grape. Other white wine grapes are Kerner (a cross between the Riesling and the red Trollinger grapes), Elbling, Ruländer (Pinot Gris), Gewürztraminer, Gutedel, Scheurebe, Ortega, Morio-Muskat and Bacchus. The black grapes include Trollinger (originally from the Tyrol), Portugieser (originating in Austria) and Spätburgunder (Pinot Noir).

There are two major categories of wine: Tafelwein (table wine) and Qualitätswein (quality wine), which is then subdivided ino QbA *(Qualitätswein bestimmter Anbaugebiete)*: quality wine in medium price range (includes Liebfraumilch) from 13 designated regions *(Anbaugebiete)*, and QmP *(Qualitätswein mit Prädikat)*: quality wines with distinction and special characteristics. They have no added sugar. The *Prädikat* describes how ripe the grape was when it was harvested—generally the riper the grape, the richer the wine. There are six categories:

1 *Kabinett*—wine is good enough to be kept in the winegrower's own cabinet.

2   *Spätlese (late harvested)*—wine is made from riper grapes to make fuller, sweeter wine.

3   *Auslese (selected harvesting)*—made from selected bunches of late-harvested grapes, these wines are even sweeter, fuller and stay longer on the palate, than Spatlese wines.

4   *Beerenauslese BA (selective picked grapes)*—wine is made from individually picked grapes which, because of their overripeness, have begun to shrivel on the vine. The resulting wine is very rich.

5   *Eiswein (ice wine)*—very sweet wines made from overripe grapes, which have been frozen by severe frosts.

6   *Trockenbeerenauslese TBA (selectively picked raisined grapes)*—Lusciously sweet wines made from shrivelled raisin-like grapes, which have been affected by *Edelfäule (Botrytis cinerea*—noble rot*)* fungus.

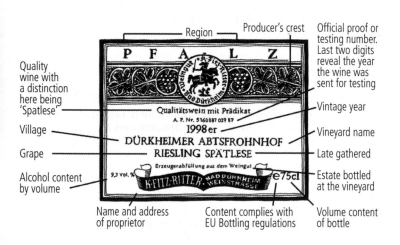

Germany has 13 specified wine-growing *Gebiete* (regions):

- Baden, Hessische Bergstrasse, Mittelrhein, Rheingau, Rheinhessen and Pfalz are all on or near the banks of the Rhine
- Franken is on the Main
- Württemberg is on the banks of the Neckar
- Mosel-Saar-Ruwer, Ahr, Nahe and Saale-Unstrut are all named after their rivers
- Sachsen vineyards are on the banks of the Elbe.

These regions contain the 39 *Bereiche* (districts), the name of which is usually taken from the best-known village of the district (e.g. Bernkastel). This is further broken down into 161 *Grosslagen* (sub-district or collective vineyard sites, e.g. Bernkasteler Badstube) and 2,644 *Einzellagen* (individual vineyard sites, e.g. Bernkasteler Doktor).

*The German wine regions (**Gebiete***) and examples of villages*

Ahr	Heimersheim, Neuenahr, Walporzheim
Baden	Michelfeld, Zulzfeld, Durbach
Franken	Castell, Iphofen, Würzburg
Heissische Bergstrasse	Bensheim, Heppenheim
Mittelrhein	Oberwesel, Boppard Hamm, Kaub, Bacharach
Mosel-Saar-Ruwer	Bernkastel-Kues, Enkirch, Erden, Graach, Kasel, Ockfen, Piesport, Wehlen, Zell
Nahe	Bad Kreuznach, Munster, Niederhausen, Schlossböckelheim
Pfalz	Bad Dürkheim, Deidesheim, Forst, Kallstadt
Rheingau	Assmannshausen, Erbach, Geisenheim, Hallgarten, Hattenheim, Hochheim, Johannisberg, Oestrich, Rauenthal, Rüdesheim, Winkel
Rheinhessen	Bingen, Oppenheim, Nierstein

Saale-Unstrut	Freyburg, Bad Kösen
Sachsen	Meissen, Radebeul, Diesbar
Württemberg	Gundelsheim, Maulbronn, Weikersheim

Greece

Best known is the famous Retsina, which is flavoured with pine-tree resin obtained from Aleppo pines in Attica. This imparts a slight turpentine flavour which many people find pleasant to taste especially with spicy foods. It is white or pink in colour and Metaxa's Retsina is a style of note. The dry white wines Demestica, Santa Helena, Antika and Pallini are light and pleasant, either as apéritifs or as accompaniments to light food. Demestica also appears as a red wine and the red Château Carras and the dark, fruity Naoussa are fast establishing good reputations. Two sweet wines, the deep golden Muscat of Samos and the intense red port-like Mavrodaphne, are popular dessert wines. More recently Greece is producing wines from the classic varietals.

Hungary

Wines are usually named after the district in which they have been made. The reds are big and burly, good foils for the heavily flavoured food. The whites are also full of personality, for the same reason. Many of the white table wines are sold simply as Hungarian Riesling or Balatoni Riesling but others are named: Badacsony, Mór, Somló, Pécs and Mecsek, usually with the grape appendage Riesling or Furmirit. Of the reds Egri Bikavér (Bull's Blood) is the most celebrated, but Kadarka, Vilány, Sopron and the ones labelled Hungarian Merlot are good-value wines.

The best known of all the wines is Tokay Aszú, a luscious golden wine produced from the Furmint and Hárslevelü grapes. Heat and dampness encourage the mould *Botrytis cinerea* (noble rot) to form on the skins. These shrink, and the grape juice becomes very concentrated as the water content is reduced and the glycerine content increases. The grapes are collected in *puttonyos* (hods)—smallish wooden barrels containing about 30 litres (8 gallons). They are then crushed to a pasty mass and added to new *must* as it ferments in a standard vat. The more *puttonyos* added, the sweeter the eventual wine. The number added will be shown on the label as either three, four, five or six *puttonyos*. The most luscious wine is called Tokay Essenz.

India

India has been making wine for centuries, with both red and white wines being produced. A well-known wine is the *méthod traditionnelle* sparkling wine, under the label Omar Khayyam, using Ugni Blanc, Pinot Blanc and Chardonnay grapes.

Israel

The Société Coopérative Vigneronne des Grandes Caves is the major producer of wine in Israel. It markets its wines under the brand name Carmel. Much of the wine is Kosher, made under Rabbinical supervision, and the main export market is to the United States. The wines range from dry to sweet, reds and whites, with some fortified and sparkling wines also made. Of the table wines, the white Cannel Hock, Château Montague, Yarden Sauvignon Blanc and Palwin are of a good standard. The best reds are Gamla Cabernet Sauvignon, Château Windsor, Adom Atic, Yarden Cabernet Sauvignon, Yarden Merlot and Golan Cabernet Sauvignon. Of the dessert wines, Yarden Late Harvested Sauvignon Blanc made from *Botrytis*-affected grapes is really fine. The better sparkling wines such as Yarden Brut, Yarden Blanc de Blancs and Gamla Rosé are made by the *méthode traditionnelle*.

Italy

Wine is grown all over Italy and is now regulated by law, although some of the very best producers operate outside the regulation laws and can now only describe their wines as table wines. The levels of quality of Italian wines are:

- **■** *Vino da tavola:* ordinary table wine, unclassified.

- **■** *Vino da tavola con indicazione geografica:* wine from a defined area.

- **■** *Denominazione de origine contrallata (DOC):* quality wine from an approved area.

- **■** *Denominazione di origine controllata e garantia (DOCG):* top classification for guaranteed quality wines from approved areas.

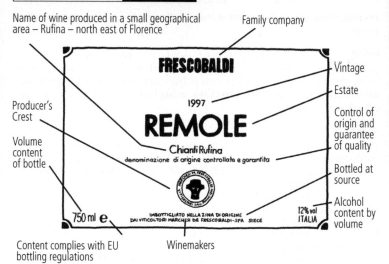

Name of wine produced in a small geographical area – Rufina – north east of Florence

Family company

Producer's Crest

Volume content of bottle

Vintage

Estate

Control of origin and guarantee of quality

Bottled at source

Alcohol content by volume

Content complies with EU bottling regulations

Winemakers

Some Italian wine terms

Abboccato	slightly sweet
Amabile	semi-sweet
Annata	vintage
Asciutto	bone dry
Bianco	white
Chiaretto	deep rosé
Classico	classical or best part of a particular wine area (e.g. Chianti Classico)
Dolce	sweet
Frizzantino	slightly sparkling

Imbottigliato da	bottled by
Nero	dark red
Riserva	matured for a specific number of years
Risenra speciale	like Riserva but older
Rosato	rosé or pink wine
Rosso	red
Secco	dry
Spumante	foaming or sparkling
Spumante Classico	sparkling wine made by the traditional method
Stravecchio	aged old wines
Vecchio	old

Piedmont

This district is the home of vermouth, which originated in Turin, the capital of Piedmont. This district is also renowned for Italy's best-known sparkling wine, Asti Spumante, with the best made from the Muscat grape and by the *Spumante Classico* method (traditional method). Cheaper varieties are produced by the *charmat* (closed tank) method. Two red wines, Barolo and Barbaresco, made from Nebbiolo grapes are really excellent, as is Barbera which is named after its own grape, and Gattinara.

Tuscany

Renowned for its red wines, Chianti Classico, Brunello di Montalcino and Vino Nobile di Montepulciano. Chianti has traditionally been made from the Sangiovese grape (although others are now permitted in the blend) and is usually sold in a globular shaped bottle *(fiasco)* which is partly covered with straw not only for appearance but, more practically, to prevent the bottles breaking when carried *en masse*. Chianti Classico wines are nowadays more usually found in Bordeaux-style bottles. The black rooster neck label is a sign of quality and the word *riserva* on a label implies that the wine has matured for five years in cask.

Trentino-Alto Adige

Wines from this region are marketed in both German and Italian. The sparkling Gran Spumante is made by the traditional method and from the Riesling and Pinot Bianco grapes. White wines include Traminer Aromatico, Terlaner, Rhine Riesling and Pinot Bianco. The reds include Lago di Caldaro, Santa Maddelena and Pinot Nero.

Umbria

The most famous white wines are Orvieto Secco (named after the cathedral city of Orvieto), which is dry, and Orvieto Abboccato or Amabile (meaning soft in the mouth), which is medium sweet. Other wines are the red and white Torgiano.

The Marches

The principal dry white wines are Verdicchio dei Castelli di Jesi and Verdicchio di Matelica. Often sold in 'waisted' bottles, they have a pale straw colour and a slightly bitter aftertaste. The principal reds are Rosso Cànero and Rosso Piceno.

Lazio

The two white wines of note here are Frascati and Est! Est!! Est!!! Frascati may be dry, medium or sweet. Est! Est!! Est!!! is either dry or has a hint of sweetness.

Campania

From the slopes of Mount Vesuvius comes the very well known Lacryma Christi (tears of Christ) which may be red, white or rosé. Greco di Tufo and Fiano di Avellino are principal whites and the reds are Ravello and Taurasi.

Sicily

Island best known for its fortified dessert wine Marsala. It is also used in Zabaglione as well as in veal and other dishes served *alla Marsala*. Sicilian table wines include Corvo (red and white) and Regaleali (red and white).

Sardinia

Island is especially noted for its sweet dessert wines such as Vernaccia di Sardegna, Moscato del Tempio, Malvasia di Sardegna and Anghelu Ruju. Table wines include the white Riviera del Corallo and the red Cannonau.

Veneto

Well known for the dry white Soave and the popular reds, Valpolicella and Bardolino. Also home of the whites, Bianco di Custoza and Verduzzo, and the sparkling Prosecco.

Emilia-Romagna

Famous for Albana di Romagna, the first white wine in all of Italy to be been given the DOCG classification. Also well known are the red, white and rosé Lambrusco Frizzante (semi-sparkling wines).

Other wine regions of Italy

Basilicata is well known for its full-bodied red wine Aglianico del Vulture. In Lombardy (around Milan), Oltrepò Pavese makes red, white, rosé and sparkling wines. Friuli Venezia Giulia is well known for two red wines Aquilea and Carso. Liguria is noted for Cinque Terra, dry or medium-sweet white wines. Abruzzi makes a good red wine Montepulciano d'Abruzzo. Molise also produces a red called Biferno. Puglia has two principal wines, the red II Falcone and the pink Rosa del Golfo. Calabria is best known for Greco di Bianco, a big, creamy sweet wine (Vino Passito). Italy's smallest wine region Val d'Aosta, produces honest wines, almost always drunk locally.

Japan

Although the climate generally is not conducive to vines, some are grown in districts that have favourable microclimates. These include Honshu, Kyushu and Hokkaido. Grapes are some of the *lambrusca* varieties but also *vinefrea* varieties including Cabernet Sauvignon, and Merlot for reds and Chardonnay and Sémillion for whites.

Lebanon

Despite all the political troubles, red and white wines continue to be made in this war-torn land. The reds are much better than the whites, being made from a blend of Cabernet Sauvignon, Syrah and Cinsault grapes. Best examples are: Château Musar and Cuvée Musar, which have good ageing qualities.

Luxembourg

Luxembourg makes quite a number of thinish white wines from grapes such as Riesling, Elbling, Gewürztraminer and Sylvaner. There is also a slightly sparkling wine called Edelperl.

Macedonia

Produces mainly red wines from the Vranac and Kratšija grapes, the deep red earthy Kratošija and Teran have the best reputations.

Malta

Cultivation of the vine is not easy in Malta where the climate can vary between torrential rain and scorching sunshine. The result is ordinary, even harsh wine. All types are made, with the Altar wine, the wine of the church, perhaps the best of all. There are pleasant dessert wines made from the Muscat grapes, and the winery Marsovin produces palatable red, white and rosé table wines. Others of note are Verdala Rosé, Lachryma Vitas (red and white), Coleiro (red and white) and the Farmers' Wine Co-operative which also produces red and white table wines.

Mexico

The home of Tequila is now getting a good reputation for wine. The best is made from varietal grapes: Cabernet Sauvignon, Barbera, Malbec, Merlot, Trebbiano, Grenache, and Zinfandel for red, and Chenin Blanc, Sauvignon Blanc, Riesling and Chardonnay for whites.

Montenegro

Produces red wines with the Vranac grape dominant. The best wine is Crnogorski Vranac.

Morocco

Plenty of red and white wines are made, with Fez and Meknes being the chief wine-producing centres. Tarik and Chante Bled, full bodied and well balanced, are typical examples. A unique wine of special interest is Gris de Boulaouane. It is a blush wine produced by the bleeding method. The grapes are suspended on sheets of white linen where they are self-pressed by their own weight. The juice slowly drips through the linen into containers and the resulting wine is aged in bottle, not in cask.

New Zealand

New Zealand is associated with some excellent table wines. The North Island, particularly Auckland and its surrounds, was the traditional homeland for the vine, but more significant vineyards are now to be found on the East Coast of the North Island in regions like Gisborne and Hawkes Bay, and on the north edge of the South Island at Marlborough.

Although the Müller Thurgau accounts for a fair amount of the production it is the Sauvignon Blanc and the Chardonnay that have enhanced New Zealand's ever growing reputation for fine white wine. Other white grapes being grown are the Rhine Riesling, Gewürztraminer, Sémillion, Pinot Blanc and Chenin Blanc. Some production is also being tried with red wines using Cabernet Sauvignon, Pinot Noir, Merlot and Pinotage vines.

Principal wineries in New Zealand include: Babich, Cloudy Bay, Collard Brothers, Cooks, Coopers Creek, Delegat's Vineyard, Hunter's Wines, Mission Vineyards, Montana Wines, Nobilo's, Penfolds Wines, Selak Wines, Te Mata Estate and the Villa Maria Estate.

Portugal

Portugal produces an array of wines from table wines to the two classic fortified wines: Port (from the Douro Valley in northern Portugal) and Madeira (from the Island of the same name). For the table wines the main quality classifications are:

■ *Vinho de mesa:* ordinary table wine, which may be a blend from several regions

■ *Vinho de meas regional:* table wine from a specified region

■ *Vinho regional:* quality wine from a particular place within a named region

- ■ *Região demarcado:* quality wines from specified regions
- ■ *Selo de garantia:* the quality and authenticity of the wine is guaranteed.

Region, name and style of wine

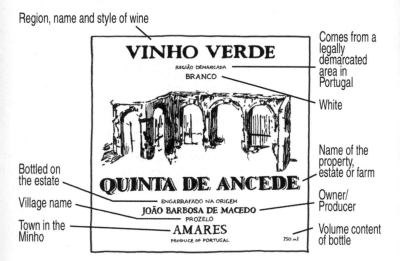

Comes from a legally demarcated area in Portugal

White

Name of the property, estate or farm

Bottled on the estate

Village name

Town in the Minho

Owner/ Producer

Volume content of bottle

Some Portuguese wine terms

Adega	winery
Coiheita	vintage
Engarrafado	bottled by
Garrafeira	wine matured in cask and bottle for some time—at least one year for white wine and two years for red wine
Quinta	estate
Região Demarcada	wine from a legally demarcated region

Reserva a quality	aged wine
Selo de Origem	seal of origin
Denominaco de Origem	guarantee of origin and quality
Vinho espumante	a sparkling wine
Vinho generoso	a strong, dessert wine

The table wines are made from a great variety of grapes in the main wine growing regions of: Bairrada, Beiras, Bucelas, Carcavelos, Colares, Dão, Estremadura, Minho, Setúbal, and Trás-os-Montes.

Bairrada

This region in the west of Portugal is known for good quality red wines which are rich in tannin when young but which, with patient ageing, become mellow and soft. White wine of average quality is made for local consumption, as are some agreeable sparkling wines. The best of the latter comes from the Quinta do Ribeirinho and is made by the *méthode traditionnelle*.

Beiras

Situated in the far north of Portugal, this area produces some rosé wines around the town of Pinhel. The region is also noted for an excellent red wine Buçaco (Bussaco) and a good *méthode traditionnelle* sparkler called Raposeira. The white wines tend to be slightly acidic.

Bucelas

Located 26 km (16 miles) north of Lisbon, this small region produces white wines from the classic Arinto grape. However, despite the noble grape, the wines are very ordinary.

Carcavelos

This is a small vine-growing area between Lisbon and Estoril. It is especially noted for its fortified almond-flavoured wine which is made at the Quinta do Barão.

Colares

These vineyards are situated by the sea about 23 km (14 miles) northwest of Lisbon. Because of the nature of the soil, the *Phylloxera* aphid could not penetrate the great carpet of sand and consequently the vineyards escaped the terrible scourge. The Ramisco grape is used to great effect in the making of Colares, producing what many consider to be the premier red wine in Portugal. In youth the wine is very astringent but age matures and mellows it out to a silky smoothness. Some undistinguished white wine is also made.

Dão

Situated in the centre of Portugal, this area is famous for its full-bodied, strong, earthy red wines. They are mostly blended and have an agreeable smoothness because of their unusually rich glycerine content. The white Dão is greatly respected and appreciated locally, but not much reaches the export market.

Estremadura

This most prolific region in all Portugal is located 115 km (70 miles) northwest of Lisbon. The red and white wines are basic table wines meant for everyday drinking. Some of the whites can have a slight effervescence.

Minho

This region produces one of the most distinctive wines in Portugal. Vinho Verde (green wine) is made close to the Spanish border but it is not a green wine as such. The 'green' refers to the youth and personality of the wine (which comes from the use of some underripe grapes) and not the colour, which is either red or white. About three times more red than white wine is made, but it is mainly the white variety that is exported.

The wines are made from grapes that are grown high up on pergolas. The grapes are picked early when they are slightly under ripe. Because of this special method of vine cultivation the grapes get less reflected sunshine, resulting in proportionally less sugar but a higher malic acid content. Once bottled, the malic acid is broken down by naturally occurring bacteria. This evolution creates a *malolactic fermentation*, which does not increase the alcohol content but produces a slight and agreeable effervescence. Vinho Verde should be drunk when it is young and vigorous. It does not require ageing.

Setúbal

Situated to the south-east of Lisbon, this area is famous for the fortified, intensely sweet, amber coloured Moscatel de Setúbal. The wine is usually aged in cask from 6 to 25 years, although younger and older examples are available. As it ages it develops an attractive honey flavour.

Trás-os-Montes

This region's name is synonymous with the internationally famous Mateus Rosé, which is beautifully labelled and presented in flagon-shaped bottles. The wine is so popular that the grape harvest of a great many vineyards in this rugged, mountainous region of the upper Douro River is given over to the production of the pink, pétillant wine.

Romania

Romanian wines have made little impact on world markets even though they are very reasonably priced. Those to look out for are the late-harvested Gewürztraminer and the Rosé Edelbeerenlese made from *botrytized* grapes. The light red Valea Lunga, the spicy red Nicoresti, the fulsome Tohani and Valea Calugareasca (Valley of the Monks) are all good with food. Last, but not least, is Cotnari, the lush white dessert wine made after the style of Tokay.

Russia and the Black Sea

With modern technology and expertise and greater awareness of the international market requirements, these wines are bound to improve. At the moment, they are on the sticky, sweet side, which suits the Russian palate well.

Moldavia, on the Romanian border, produces Negru de Purkar, a high-strength red wine with good ageing potential. It is made from the Cabernet Sauvignon, Saperavi and Rara Neagra grapes. Fetjaska is the principal grape for white wines.

Massandra in the Crimea is the dessert wine centre using mainly the Muscatel grape. Good sparkling wines, such as Kaffla and Krim, are made by the *méthode traditionnelle*. Georgia, with its vineyards in the valley of the River Rion, makes decent red wines like Mukuzani and Saperavi and straw-coloured whites Tsinandal and Rkatiseli. Some sparkling wine is made and marketed as Champanski. Russia produces mainly white and sparkling wine from around Krosnador. Stavropol, east of Krosnador, makes dryish white as well as the good dessert wine Muscatel Praskoveiski. In Armenia, port-style and sherry-style wines are made as well as table wines like the red Norashen, the white Echmiadzin and the pink Pamid. Perla (white) and Iskra (red) are the sparklers.

Serbia

Makes red, white and rosé wines. The reds and rosés are made mostly from the Prokupac grape, Smederevka is the principal white grape. The better vineyards are located around Zupa, south of Belgrade, but many of the best white wines come from grapes grown on the cool hillsides of Fruska Gora. Kosova also has dry to sweetish red wines, made from the Pinot Noir grape, which sell under the brand name Amselfeld (German for Kosova).

Slovenia

The white wine-producing Slovenia has Ljutomer, Maribor and Ptuz as the commercial centres. Lutomer Riesling is the best-known wine, followed by Lutomer Welschriesling (Lash Riesling) and the sweet Spätlese wine Ranina Radgona (tiger's milk). There is also a small amount of Renski Riesling made using, as the name suggests, the Rhine Riesling grape.

South Africa

The best white wines of South Africa come from the areas around Stellenbosch, Paarl and Tulbagh, with Riesling, Sauvignon Blanc, Clairette Blanche and Steen the favoured grapes. Owing to the hot climate the wines undergo a slow, temperature-controlled fermentation to preserve quality. South African white wines are lively and refreshing and intended to be drunk young. Good examples are: Fleur du Cap Sauvignon Blanc, Twee Jongegezellen, KWV Chenin Blanc, Theuniskraal

Riesling Groot Constantia Gewürztraminer, Zonnebloem Noble Late Harvest Superior.

South African red wines are mainly produced in Constantia, Durbanville, Paarl and Stellenbosch, where Cabernet Sauvignon, Shiraz., Gamay, Pinot Noir and Pinotage (Pinot Noir and Cinsault cross) are the most used grapes. South African reds may be light- or full-bodied. Examples include: Zonnebloem Cabernet Sauvignon, KWV Roodeberg, Culemborg Pinotage, Château Libertas, Nederburg Cabernet, Backsberg Estate.

For both the red and the white wines, most bottles show a coloured seal of origin known locally as the 'bus ticket': blue guarantees the location of production; red guarantees that at least 75 per cent of the wine was made in the year indicated on the label; green certifies that at least 75 per cent of the wine was made from the indicated grape; and gold suggests a wine of superior quality.

South Africa also makes the sherry-style wines particularly the fino variety. The best finos come from Stellenbosch and Paarl and are matured by the solera system. The sweeter sherries-style wines are made in Worcester, Robertson, Montagu and Bonnievale, areas which also produce dessert wines such as the Muscatels and many styles of port.

The Oude Meester Company make a fine brandy called Oude Meester (Old Master) and the best-known liqueur from South Africa is the tangerine flavoured Van der Hum, meaning 'What's its name?'.

Spain

Spain has the largest area of vineyards in the world and produces excellent wine in a wide variety of styles. Nearly all the best table wine of Spain come under the Denominación de Origen (DO) laws. Denominación de Origen Calificada is the super category indicating the finest quality wines.

Some Spanish wine terms

Abocado	medium sweet
Año	year
Blanco	white

Bodega	winery
Cava	cellar or generic name for sparkling wine made by the metodo tradicional
Clarete	light red table wine
Cosecha	vintage
Consejo Regulado	regulating body—stamp on the label ensures authenticity
Embotellado por	bottled by
Espumoso	sparkling
Gran reserva	red wines which have aged for at least two years in oak casks and three years in the bottle; white and rosé wines aged for at least four years including at least six months in oak casks.
Reserva	red wines which have aged for at least one year in oak casks and two years in the bottle; white and rosé wines aged for at least two years including six months in oak casks.
Rosado	rosé, pink
Seco	dry
Semi-seco	medium dry
Sin crianza	without wood age
Tinto	red
Vendimia	vintage harvest
Viña	vineyard
Vino de mesa	ordinary table wine

Of all the wines produced sherry is the most famous. This fortified wine is produced in southern Spain in the Province of Cadiz. The vineyards are

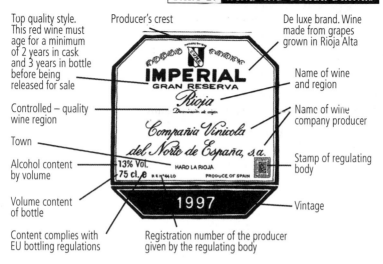

Top quality style. This red wine must age for a minimum of 2 years in cask and 3 years in bottle before being released for sale

Producer's crest

De luxe brand. Wine made from grapes grown in Rioja Alta

Name of wine and region

Controlled – quality wine region

Name of wine company producer

Town

Alcohol content by volume

Stamp of regulating body

Volume content of bottle

Vintage

Content complies with EU bottling regulations

Registration number of the producer given by the regulating body

situated around three towns, Jerez de la Frontera, Sanlúcar de Barrameda and Puerto de Santa Maria. The two grapes used are Listan (Palomino) and Pedro Ximénez (PX). Whereas sherry is produced in the south, most of the finer table wines are produced in the north in regions such as Rioja and Catalonia.

Rioja

Tempranillo, Garnacha, Graciano and Mazuelo grapes produce Spain's famous red wines. The Rio Oja, a tributary of the Ebro, gives its name to the locality which is divided into three regions: Rioja Alta (the best Rioja area), Alavesa (the next best) and Rioja Baja. The wines are big, soft, rich and mellow with a distinctive oaky flavour derived from being matured in small 225-litre oak casks for up to six years. Best examples are Marqués de Murrieta, Marqués de Riscal, Marqués de Cáceres, Viña Tondonia, la Rioja Alta, of which the style Viña Ardanza Reserva 904 is quite outstanding, and CVNE (Compania Vinicola del North de Espana).

Some good white Riojas from Malvasia and Viura grapes are also made, such as Marqués de Cáceres, Marqués de Murrieta, Viña Soledad and CVNE.

Penedès

Excellent sparkling and still white and red wines are made here. The sparkling variety is sold under the generic name of *cava* (cellar). Made by the *metodo tradicional*, it is widely available under proprietary brand names such as Gran Codornu, Freixenet Cordon Negro, Segura Viudas and Castellblanch Brut Zero.

The white wines of Penedès are a revelation especially Torres Gran Viña Sol Green Label made from Parellada and Sauvignon Blanc grapes. Torres also makes Viña Esmeralda, a medium-sweet wine made from Muscat and Gewürztraminer grapes. The dry, crisp Jean León Chardonnay and Marqués de Ailela are produced near the suburbs of Barcelona. Of the red wines, Torres again produces the pedigree wines Gran Coronas (Cabernet Sauvignon and Tempranillo) and Grand Coronas Black Label (Cabernet Sauvignon and Cabernet Franc). Jean León's Cabernet Sauvignon is also excellent.

Ribera del Duero

Ribera del Duero produces, in small quantities, the great classic red, Vega Sicilia Unico Reserva—a wine that ages well up to 30 years and is considered one of the finest reds in the world. It is made from the Cabernet Sauvignon, Malbec and Merlot grapes and is expensive. Tinto Valbuena is another fine, slightly less expensive, wine produced in the same bodega near Valladolid. Look out for Bodega Alejandro Fernandez Tinta Pesquera and Bodega Hermanos Perez Viña Pedrosa, which offer good value.

Other wine-producing regions

Navarra

The region of Navarra is located on the border of Rioja and spills over into Rioja Baja. The red, white and rosé wines get heavy media promotion as alternatives to Rioja, but they are robust by comparison. Watch for the names Bodegas Villafranca Monte Ory Reserva, Julián

Chivite Gran Feudo Tinto, Agro Navarra Camponuevo Tinto, Señorío de Sarrla Viña Ecoyen Tinto and Viña del Perdon Tinto.

Andalucia
This region produces a lovely fortified dessert wine, Málaga, once known as 'Mountain', that is rarely seen nowadays outside Spain. Made from the Pedro Ximénez and Muscat grapes, it undergoes the blending and maturing process of the solera. The best style is Lágrima ('tear', as in 'weep') made from grapes which are self-pressed by their own weight. Bodegas Barcelo and Scholtz Hennanos make quality Málaga.

La Mancha
The Midi of Spain produces large quantities of table wines. Valdepeñas (Valley of Stones) produces sound red and white wines which are used in and around Madrid.

Alicante
This region is best known for its rosé and for the extremely dark red Vino de Doble Pasta made by adding a double quantity of grape skins, which deeply darkens the colour during fermentation.

Ampurdán (Costa Brava)
This area is best known for its sparkling wine, Perelada, which is made by the *metodo tradicional*.

Switzerland

The quality of Swiss wine is consistently good. The country is made up of 25 *cantons* (districts), most of which produce wine. The three main wine regions are The French-speaking cantons (the largest wine area), the Italian-speaking cantons and the German-speaking cantons.

French-speaking cantons

The three main wine areas are: Valais, The Vaud, Geneva and Neuchâtel.

Valais
The Valais wine-growing area extends along the entire valley of the Rhône from Viège to Martigny. The region produces good red and white wines. The red Dôle is made from Gamay and Pinot Noir grapes. Petite Dôle is a red wine made solely from Pinot Noir grapes. Of the whites,

Fendant made from the Chasselas grapes is best, but there are other good styles such as the Johannisberg. Vin du Glacier is a white wine made in the Anniviers Valley and then taken to caves in the mountains near the glaciers to mature in larch-wood casks for up to 15 years. Malvoisie is an estate-bottled, straw-coloured, dessert wine made from late-gathered noble rot grapes.

The Vaud

Vaud vineyards are located along the shores of Lake Geneva (Lac Léman) and include three smaller districts: La Côte, Lavaux and Chablais. The area is generally known for its fine white wines made from the Chasselas (Dorm locally) grape. Prime examples are Dézaley, Mont-sur-Rolle, Saint Saphorin and Aigle Clos de Murailles. The latter is one of the finest and most expensive of all Swiss wines.

Geneva

Adjoining the Vaud are the vineyards of Geneva. Half the white wine production is from the Chasselas grape with other white grapes being the Aligoté and Chardonnay. Red wines are made from the Gamay grape.

Neuchâtel

Neuchâtel produces light fragrant white wines mostly from the Chasselas grape. Some are pétillant and produce the famous Neuchâtel Star when poured from a height into the glass. There is also a red Pinot Noir wine called Cortaillod and a pink one called Oeil de Perdrix (partridge eye) made from the same grape.

German-speaking cantons

The main wine regions here are situated near the German border in an area known as Ostschweiz (east Switzerland). White wines are mainly from Riesling-Sylvaner (Müller Thurgau), and the reds from Blauburgunder (Pinot Noir), also know as Clevner of Beerli. Elsewhere there are examples of wines made from Chardonnay and Pinot Noir.

Italian-speaking cantons

Wines here are made in southern Switzerland with mainly red wines made from the Merlot grape, and sometimes blended with Cabernet Sauvignon. A small amount of white wine is made from the Chasselas, Sémillion and Sauvignon Blanc grapes.

Tunisia

The vineyards are located in the north, with mostly red and rosé wines being produced from the Alicante Bouchet, Carignan, Cabernet Sauvignon, Mourvèdre and Grenache grapes. Whites are made from Clairette and Ugni Blanc grapes, with a big strong dessert wine being made from the Muscat grape.

Turkey

Much of the grape production in Turkey is used for table grapes and sultanas, but some reasonable wine is also made. The majority of the wine is red, good examples being Villa Doluca, Hosbag, Buzbag and Trakya Kirmisi. The dry Trakya made from the Sémillon grape is the best of the whites.

United States of America

The majority of States cultivate the vine for making wine. Of these, California is the prime region producing the vast majority of the wine. Other principal States are New York State, Washington State and its neighbour Oregon, Texas and Maryland.

There two qualities of wine made in the United States: Table wines and Premium wines:

Table wines

These are popular reliable, attractive, inexpensive and made in huge quantities by the ultra-modern, fully automated wineries. Technically sound, the wines are blended to a recipe. We would call them carafe wines. In America they are known as 'Jug wines' as they are traditionally sold by the jug-full in diners and restaurants throughout the country.

Premium wines

These are the best quality and are made by proprietors working on a smaller scale. These designer wines are crafted to the highest standard in boutique wineries especially in California. Many of the wine growers are graduates of the Wine College of the University of California at Davis. These masters of cultured yeast, use meticulous control of fermentation temperatures and technical innovations to help nature in making good wines great. They are now producing wines of real quality, concentrating on elegance and subtlety rather than on alcohol and powerfully dominating flavours. Sparkling wines are also made by the traditional method, closed tank method or the transfer method, and are sometimes labelled as Champagne, which they are not.

The USA also has a form of appellation known as Approved Viticultural Areas (AVAs). Briefly it stipulates that:

- Varietal wines must use a minimum of 75 per cent of the grape named on the label;
- When a geographic source is indicated, at least 75 per cent of the wine must come from there;
- Wines from a specific vintage or from a nominated particular estate, must have at least 95 per cent of that wine in the bottle.

However, not all wineries adhere to these constrictions. They blend in whatever proportions suit their needs. Basically there are two qualities of wine made in the United States.

California

With its benign climate, accommodating soil and ideal aspects, California is a natural home for the vine. Many of the vineyard sites are also blessed by a unique microclimate. The Californian coastal fog shrouds the vines throughout the summer from the fierce morning sunrays. This benefits the quality of the grapes by slowing down and prolonging the ripening process. The main grapes used are the European varieties Cabernet Sauvignon, Pinot Noir and Merlot as well as the indigenous Zinfandel for red wines. The Chardonnay, Sauvignon Blanc (Fumé Blanc) and Johannisberg Riesling are the principal white grapes in use. The major areas of production are the classic Napa Valley and the Sonoma Valley, Mendocino and the central coast from Monterey to Santa Barbara.

Wines are marketed under the names of the producers. These include: Acacia, Alexander Valley, Almadén, Beaulieu, Beringer, Boeger, Buena Vista, Callaway, Ch. Montelena, Ch. St Jean, Chalone, Clos du Bois, Clos du Val, Concannon Vineyard, Domaine Chandon, Dry Creek, Edna

Valley, Fetzer, Firestone Vineyard, Freemark Abbey, Gallo, Hanzell, Heitz Cellars (Martha's Vineyard and Bella Oaks), Inglenook, Iron Horse, Jekel, Jordan, Joseph Phelps, Kahlin, Korbel, Mantanzas Creek, Mark West, Mayacamas, Monticello, Mumm Napa, Paul Masson, Piper Sonoma, Preston, Ravenswood, Ridge Vineyards, Robert Mondavi, Roederer Estate, Rubicon, Rutherford Hill, Saintsbury, Sanford, Schramsberg, Simi, Stags Leap, Sterling Vineyards, Stevenot, Storybook, The Christian Brothers, Trefethen, Wente and Wild Horse.

New York State

Traditionally, the New York wine industry was based on the use of *Vitis labrusca* vines (Concord, Catawba, Delaware, Dutchess, Ives and Niagara). The *labrusca* vines were chosen initially to withstand the arctic conditions of winter. Later it was discovered that other species could also cope with the extremes of climate. Hybrids based on *labrusca* and *vinifera* vines (Vidal Blanc, Seyval Blanc, Chelois, Baco Noir, De Chaunac, Aurore, Maréchal Foch) have been developed. More recently the classic vinifera vines have also been successfully planted. The main areas of production are Finger Lakes, Long Island and the Hudson River Valley.

Finger Lakes

Here *Vitis labrusca* hybrids and *Vitis vinifera* vines are grown to produce grapes for wine. The current trend is to use the classic *vinifera* vines with the white Chardonnay, Riesling and Gewürztraminer proving particularly successful. Splendid sparkling wine, made by the classical method, is a feature of the region. Prime brands are Gold Seal, Great Western and Taylor.

Long Island

Wineries in Long Island are concentrating more and more on *Vitis vinifera* vines and are now successfully cultivating Merlot, Cabernet Sauvignon and Cabernet Franc for red wines, and Chardonnay and Sauvignon Blanc for whites. Most of the wineries are situated in the North Fork Peninsula.

Hudson River Valley

This is the oldest wine region in New York State. Here the hybrid Seyval Blanc reigns supreme, but the current vogue is for *vinifera* vines Cabernet

Sauvignon and Pinot Noir for red wines and Chardonnay and Riesling for white wines. Benmarl Wine Company, Clinton Vineyards, Millbrook Vineyards and the Rivendell Winery have all established good reputations.

Oregon

Oregon's vineyards are concentrated in the Willamette Valley, Umpqua Valley and Rogue Valley. Although the general climatic conditions are cool, the coast range in the west and the Cascade Mountains in the east prevent them from being extreme. Mostly *Vitis vinifera* vines are cultivated: Chardonnay, Müller-Thurgau, Sauvignon Blanc and Pinot Gris for white wines, and Pinot Noir, Merlot and Cabernet Sauvignon for reds.

Washington State

With a hot, arid climate, irrigation is necessary. The sweltering summer days are counterbalanced by cool temperatures at night so the grapes have a healthy acidity. *Vitis vinifera* vines were first introduced in the 1950s. Chardonnay, Sauvignon Blanc, Sémillon for white wine, and Cabernet Sauvignon and Merlot for reds are all cultivated successfully. The main vineyards are grouped in Yakima Valley, Columbia Valley, Walla Walla Valley and Spokane. Château Ste Michelle, Associated Vintners, Hinzerling, Preston Wine Cellars, the Hogue Cellars and Leonetti Cellar are the best-known producers.

Texas

With its extreme, arid, climate it is hard to imagine Texas as being vine friendly. Yet, due to modern, sophisticated irrigation, which uses the drip method to water each vine individually, the grape has been successfully cultivated. Texas produces over 1 million cases of wine annually and is now the fourth largest wine-producing state in the United States. The three major areas of production are the High Plains near Lubbock, Austin in the Hill Country and West Texas. Mostly *vinifera* vines are cultivated Sauvignon Blanc, Chenin Blanc and Chardonnay for whites and Pinot Noir and Zinfandel for reds.

Maryland

Wines to look out for are, Chardonnay for white wines and Cabernet Sauvignon for red wines. Other grapes for white wines also include Riesling.

NON-ALCOHOLIC DRINKS

Aerated waters

These are drinks that are charged or aerated with carbonic gas. Artificial aerated waters are by far the most common. The flavourings found in different aerated waters are imparted from various essences. Some examples of these aerated waters are:

- Soda water: colourless and tasteless
- Tonic water: colourless and quinine flavoured
- Dry ginger: golden straw coloured with a ginger flavour
- Bitter lemon: pale cloudy coloured with a sharp lemon flavour

Other flavoured waters, which come under this heading, are:

- 'Fizzy' lemonades
- Orangeaid
- Ginger beer
- Coca-cola, etc.

Natural spring waters/mineral waters

The EU has divided bottled water into two main types: mineral water and spring water. *Mineral water* has a mineral content (which is strictly controlled), while *spring water*, obtained from natural springs, has fewer regulations, apart from those concerning hygiene. Water can be still, naturally sparkling or carbonated during bottling.

Examples of mineral waters

Appollinaris	Naturally sparkling	Germany
Contrex	Still	France
Perrier	Naturally sparkling and also in fruit flavours	France
Royal Farris	Naturally sparkling	Norway
San Pellegrino	Carbonated	Italy
Spa	Still, naturally sparkling or in fruit flavours	Belgium
Spa Monopole	Still or sparkling	Belgium
Vichy Celestines	Naturally sparkling	France
Vittel	Naturally sparkling	France
Volvic	Still	France

Examples of spring waters

Ashbourne	Still or sparkling	England
Badoit	Slightly sparkling	France
Buxton	Still or carbonated	England
Evian	Still	France
Highland Spring	Still or carbonate	Scotland
Malvern	Still or carbonated	England

Squashes

Squashes may be served on their own, mixed with spirits or cocktails, or used as the base for such drinks as fruit cups. They are indispensable in the bar and an adequate stock should always be held. Examples are:

- orange
- lemon squash
- grapefruit
- lime juice

Juices

The main types of juices are:

Bottled or canned

- orange juice
- pineapple juice
- grapefruit juice
- tomato juice

Fresh

- orange
- grapefruit
- lemon
- pineapple

Syrups

The main use of these concentrated, sweet, fruit flavourings is as a base for cocktails, fruit cups or mixed with soda water as a long drink. The main ones used are:

- grenadine (pomegranate)
- cassis (blackcurrant)
- citronelle (lemon)
- gomme (white sugar syrup)
- framboise (raspberry)
- cerise (cherry)
- orgeat (almond)

Syrups are also available as 'flavouring agents' for cold milk drinks such as milk shakes.

ALCOHOLIC DRINKS

Bitters

Bitters are used either as apéritifs or for flavouring mixed drinks and cocktails. The most popular varieties are:

Amer Picon

This is a black and bitter French apéritif. Grenadine or Cassis is often added to make the flavour more acceptable. Traditionalists add water in a proportion 2:1.

Angostura bitters

Takes its name from a town in Bolivia. However, it is no longer produced there but in Trinidad. Brownish red in colour, it is used in the preparation of pink gin and the occasional cocktail and may be regarded as mainly a flavouring agent.

Byrrh

(Pronounced beer.) This is a style of bitters made in France near the Spanish border. It has a base of red wine and is flavoured with quinine and herbs and fortified with brandy.

Campari

A pink, bitter-sweet Italian apéritif that has a slight flavour of orange peel and quinine.

Fernet Branca

Italian version of Amer Picon. Best served diluted with water or soda. Good for hangovers!

Underberg

German bitter which looks, and almost tastes, like iodine. It may be taken as a pick-me-up with soda.

Other bitters

Orange and peach bitters are used principally as cocktail ingredients.

Alcoholic strength

Three scales of measurement

The main scale of measurement of alcoholic strength may be summarised as:

- OIML Scale (European): range 0 per cent to 100 per cent (percentage by volume)

- Sikes Scale (United Kingdom old scale): range 0° to 175° ('Proof' was the point 100°). 70° proof is equal to 40 per cent alcohol by volume.

- American Scale (USA): range 0° to 200°. Similar to Sikes but has scale of 0° to 200° rather than 0° to 175°.

The percentage by volume measurement indicates the amount of pure alcohol in a liquid. Thus a liquid measured as 40 per cent alcohol by volume will have 40 per cent of the contents as pure alcohol. The alcoholic content of drinks, as percentage by volume, is now almost always shown on labels.

Approximate alcoholic strengths of drinks

- not more that 0.05 per cent   alcohol free
- not more than 0.5 per cent   de-alcoholised
- up to 1.2 per cent   low alcohol
- 3–6 per cent   beer, cider, FABs[1] and 'alcopops'[2] with any of these being up to 10 per cent
- 8–15 per cent   wines, usually around 10–13 per cent
- 14–22 per cent   fortified wines (liqueur wines) such as sherry and port, aromatised wines such as vermouth, vin doux naturels such as Muscat de Beaumes-de-Venise and Sake[3]
- 37.5–45 per cent   spirits, usually at 40 per cent
- 17–55 per cent   liqueurs, very wide range

[1] 'FAB': 'flavoured alcoholic beverages' e.g. 'Barcardi Breezer' (5.4 per cent)

[2] 'alcopops': manufactured flavoured drinks (generally sweet and fruity), which have had alcohol, such as gin, added to them. They are also known as alcoholic soft drinks or alcoholic lemonade. Usually 3.5 to 5 per cent but can be up to 10 per cent.

[3] 'Sake': strong (18 per cent), slightly sweet, form of beer made from rice.

Other bitters are Appenzeller, Amora Montenegro, Radis, Unicum, Abbots, Peychaud, Boonekamp, Welling and Weisflog. Many are used to cure that 'morning after the night before' feeling. Cassis or Grenadine are sometimes added to make the drink more palatable.

Fortified wines

Fortified wines such as Sherry and Port, have been strengthened by the addition of alcohol, usually a grape spirit. These are now known within the EU as liqueur wines or *vin de liqueur*. Their alcoholic strength may be between 15 per cent and *22 per cent,* by volume.

- Sherry (from Spain) 15–18 per cent—Fino (dry), Almacenista (old unblended) Manzanilla (type of fino), Amontillado (medium), Palo Cortado (between Amontillado and Oloroso), Oloroso (sweet)

- Port (from Portugal) 18–22 per cent—Wood Port: white, ruby, and tawny. Bottle Port: crusted, late bottled vintage (LBV), vintage character and vintage

- Madeira 18 per cent (made on the Portuguese island of Madeira)— Sercial (dry), Verdelho (medium), Bual (sweet), Malmsey (very sweet)

- Málaga 18–20 per cent—made in similar way to port and comes from the Province of Málaga, Andalusia, Spain

- Marsala 18 per cent—a dark sweet wine from Marsala in Sicily

Aromatised wines

These are flavoured and fortified wines

Vermouths

These come in four main types:

- Dry vermouth: often called French vermouth or simply French. It is made from dry white wine that is flavoured and fortified.

- Sweet vermouth/bianco: made from dry white wine, flavoured, fortified and sweetened with sugar or mistelle.

- Rosé vermouth: made in a similar way to Bianco but it is less sweet and is coloured with caramel.

■ Red vermouth: often called Italian vermouth, Italian or more often It (as in Gin and It). It is made from white wine and is flavoured, sweetened and coloured with a generous addition of caramel.

Key trade names are: Chambery, Martini, Cinzano and Noilly Prat.

Chamberyzette

Made in the Savoy Alps of France. It is flavoured with the juice of wild strawberries.

Punt-e-mes

From Carpano of Turin; this is heavily flavoured with quinine and has wild contrasts of bitterness and sweetness.

Dubonnet

Dubonnet is available in two varieties: blonde (white) and rouge (red) and is flavoured with quinine and herbs.

St Raphael

Red or white, bitter-sweet drink from France flavoured with herbs and quinine.

Lillet

Popular French apéritif made from white Bordeaux wine and flavoured with herbs, fruit peel and fortified with Armagnac brandy. It is aged in oak casks.

Pineau des Charentes

Although not strictly an aromatised or fortified wine, *Pineau des Charentes* has gained popularity as an alternative apéritif or digestif. It is available in white, amber or rosé and is made with grape must from the Cognac region and fortified with young Cognac to about 17 per cent alcohol by volume. Also called a *mistelle*.

Spirits

Spirits are produced by the distillation of alcoholic beverages. The principle of distillation is that ethyl alcohol vaporizes (boils) at a lower temperature (78°C) than water (100°C). Thus where a liquid containing alcohol is heated in an enclosed environment the alcohol will form steam first and can be taken off, leaving water and other ingredients behind. This process raises the alcoholic strength of the resulting liquid. There are two main methods of producing spirits, either by the pot still method, which is used for full, heavy flavoured spirits such as brandy, or the patent still (Coffey) method, which produces the lighter spirits such as vodka.

Aquavit

Made in Scandinavia from potatoes or grain and flavoured with herbs, mainly caraway seeds. To be appreciated fully, Aquavit must be served chilled.

Arrack

Made from the sap of palm trees. The main countries of production are Java, India, Ceylon and Jamaica.

Brandy terms	
*	3 years maturing in cask
**	4 years in cask
***	5 years in cask
VO	(very old) 10–12 years in cask
VSO	(very superior or special old) 12–17 years in cask
VSOP	(very superior or special old pale) 20–25 years in cask
VVSOP	(very very superior or special old pale) 40 years in cask
XO	up to 45 years in cask
Extra	70 years in cask
Fine Maison	brandy of the house
Fine Champagne	Cognac made from Grande and Petite Champagne grown grapes
Grande Fine Champagne	Cognac made only from Grande Champagne grapes

Brandy

Brandy may be defined as a spirit distilled from wine. The word brandy is more usually linked with the names Cognac and Armagnac, but brandy is also made in almost all wine producing areas.

Eau de vie

Fermented and distilled juice of fruit. Much of the best comes from the Alsace area of France, Germany, Switzerland and Yugoslavia. Examples are:

- Himbergeist from wild raspberries (Germany)
- Kirschwasser (Kirsch) from cherries (Germany)
- Mirabelle from plums (France)
- Quetsch from plums (Alsace and Germany)
- Poire William from pears (Switzerland and Alsace)
- Slivovitz from plums (Yugoslavia)
- Fraise from strawberries (France, especially Alsace)
- Framboise from raspberries (France, especially Alsace)

Gin

Gets its name from the first part of the word Genièvre, which is the French term for juniper. Juniper is the principal botanical (flavouring agent) used in the production of gin. The word Geneva is the Dutch translation of the botanical, juniper. Maize is the cereal used in gin production in the United Kingdom, however, rye is the main cereal generally used in the production of Geneva gin and other Dutch gins. Malted barley is an alternative. The two key ingredients (botanicals) used for flavouring are juniper berries and coriander seeds. Types of gin are:

- Fruit gins: fruit flavoured gins that may be produced from any fruit. The most popular are sloe, orange and lemon.

- Geneva gin: Made in Holland by the pot still method alone and is generally known as 'Hollands' gin.

- London Dry Gin: Most well-known and popular of all the gins. It is unsweetened.

- Old Tom: Gin made' in Scotland and sweetened with sugar syrup. Traditionally used in a Tom Collins cocktail.
- Plymouth Gin: Stonger flavour than London Dry and most well known for its use in the cocktail Pink Gin, together with the addition of Angostura Bitters.

Grappa

Italian style brandy produced from the pressings of grapes after the required must unfermented grape juice has been removed for wine production. It is similar in style to the French marc brandy.

Marc

Local French brandy made where wine is grown. Usually takes the name of the region, e.g. Marc de Borgogne.

Mirabelle

Colourless spirit made from plums. The main country of origin is France.

Pastis

Name given to spirits flavoured with anis and/or liquorice, such as Pernod. The spirit is made in many Mediterranean countries and is popular almost everywhere. It has taken over from the infamous absinthe, once known as the 'Green Goddess'. The latter has since been banned in France.

Quetsch

Colourless spirit with plums being the main ingredient. The key countries of production are the Balkans, France and Germany. It has a brandy base.

Rum

Spirit made from the fermented by-products of sugar cane. It is produced in countries where sugar cane grows naturally and is available in dark and light varieties.

Schnapps

Spirit distilled from a fermented potato base and flavoured with caraway seed.

Tequila

Mexican spirit distilled from the fermented juice of the agave plant. It is traditionally drunk after a lick of salt and a squeeze of lime or lemon.

Vodka

A highly rectified (very pure) pâtént still spirit. It is purified by being passed through activated charcoal which removes virtually all aroma and flavour. It is described as a colourless and flavourless spirit.

Whisk(e)y

Whisky or whiskey is a spirit made from cereals: Scotch whisky from malted barley, Irish whiskey usually from barley, North American whiskey and Bourbon from maize and rye. The spelling whisky usually refers to the Scotch or Canadian drink and whiskey to the Irish or American.

- Scotch whisky is primarily made from barley, malted (hence the term malt whisky) then heated over a peat fire. Grain whiskies are made from other grains and are usually blended with malt whisky.

- Irish whiskey differs from Scotch in that hot air rather than peat fire is used during malting, thus Irish does not gain the smoky quality of Scotch. It is also distilled three times (rather than two as in the making of Scotch) and is matured longer.

- Canadian whisky is usually a blend of flavoured and neutral whiskies made from grains such as rye, wheat and barley.

- American whiskey is made from various mixtures of barley, maize and rye. Bourbon is made from maize.

- Japanese whisky is made by the Scotch process and is blended.

Liqueurs

Liqueurs are defined as sweetened and flavoured spirits. They should not be confused with liqueur spirits, which may be whiskies or brandies of

Popular liqueurs

Name	Colour	Flavour/spirit base	Country
Abricotine	Red	Apricot/brandy	France
Avocaat	Yellow	Egg, sugar/brandy	Holland
Anisette	Clear	Aniseed/neutral spirit	France, Spain, Italy, Holland
Amaretto	Golden	Almonds	Italy
Archers	Clear	Peaches/Schnapps	UK
Arrack	Clear	Herbs, sap of palm trees	Java, India, Sri Lanka, Jamaica
Bailey's Irish Cream	Coffee	Honey, chocolate, cream, whiskey	Ireland
Benedictine Dom	Yellow/green	Herbs/brandy	France
Calvados	Amber	Apple/brandy	France
Chartreuse	Green (45 per cent abv) Yellow (55 per cent abv)	Herbs, plants/brandy	France
Cherry Brandy	Deep red	Cherry/brandy	Denmark
Cointreau	Clear	Orange/brandy	France
Crème de cacao	Dark brown	Chocolate, vanilla/rum	France
Drambuie	Golden	Heather, honey, herbs/whisky	Scotland
Galliano	Golden	Herbs/berries/flowers/roots	Italy
Grand Marnier	Amber	Orange/brandy	France
Glayva	Golden	Herbs, spice/whisky	Scotland
Kirsch	Clear	Cherry/neutral spirit	Alsace
Kahlúa	Pale chocolate	Coffee/rum	Mexico
Kümmel	Clear	Caraway seed/neutral spirit	East European countries
Malibu	Clear	Coconut/white rum	Caribbean
Maraschino	Clear	Maraschino cherry	Italy
Parfait amour	Violet	Violets, lemon peel, spices	France/Holland
Sambuca	Clear	Liquorice/neutral spirit	Italy
Slivovitz	Clear	Plum/brandy	East Europe
Southern Comfort	Golden	Peaches/oranges/whiskey	United States
Strega (The witch)	Yellow	Herbs/bark/fruit	Italy
Tia Maria	Brown	Coffee/rum	Jamaica
Van der hum	Amber	Tangerine/brandy	South Africa

great age and quality. For instance, a brandy liqueur is a liqueur with brandy as a basic ingredient, whilst a liqueur brandy may be defined as a brandy of great age and excellence. Liqueurs are made by two basic methods:

- Heat or infusion method: best when herbs, peels, roots, etc are being used as heat can extract the oils, flavours and aromas
- Cold or maceration method: best when soft fruits are used to provide the flavours and aromas

The heat method uses a pot still for distillation purposes whilst the cold method allows the soft fruit to soak in brandy in oak casks over a long period of time.

Beer

Beer in one form or another is an alcoholic beverage found in all bars and areas dispensing alcoholic beverages. Beers are fermented drinks, deriving their alcoholic content from the conversion of malt sugars, made using various grains, into alcohol by brewers yeast, and being flavoured with hops. The alcoholic content of beer varies according to type, usually between 3.5–10 per cent alcohol by volume.

Cider

Cider is an alcoholic beverage obtained through the fermentation of apple juice, or a mixture of apple juice and up to 25 per cent pear juice. Draught cider, which is dull in appearance, may be completely dry (known in the UK as 'scrumpy'), or sweetened with sugar. Key and bottled ciders are pasteurised or sterile filtered to render them star-bright and they may be sweetened. It may also undergo a second fermentation, usually in a tank, to make sparkling cider or may be carbonated.

Perry

Perry is an alcoholic beverage obtained through the fermentation of pear juice, or a mixture of pear and apple juice and up to 25 per cent. It is usually sparkling and may be carbonated or the sparkle may come from a second fermentation in sealed tanks. In the production of perry the processes of filtering, blending and sweetening are all carried out under pressure.

Examples of common drinks and their service

Drink	Service
Baileys	Either chilled or with crushed ice as frappé
Brandy	No additions to good brandies. Popular mixers for lesser brandies are lemonade or peppermint, together with ice
Campari	Soda water or lemonade together with ice and slice of orange
Dark Rum	Lemonade or cola with ice and slice of lemon/lime or with blackcurrant and no ice
Sherries	Serve chilled
Fruit Juices	Served chilled or serve with lemonade, tonic water, or sparkling mineral water, also served with ice and a slice of lemon or orange or other fruit
Gin	Angostura Bitters and ice (Pink Gin) or with tonic water or bitter lemon together with ice and slice of lemon/lime
Liqueurs	May be served naturally or on crushed ice as frappé
Mineral water	Properly served chilled only, but can be with ice and lemon/lime at the request of the guest. Sometimes served with cordials or fruit juices
Aerated waters (e.g. cola)	Served chilled or with ice, and slice of lemon/lime or orange. Sometimes served with cordials
Pernod	Water and with ice offered and sometimes with cordials or lemonade
Pimm's	Lemonade, ice and slice of lemon, cucumber, apple, orange and a sprig of mint. Sometimes also topped up with ginger ale or soda or tonic water
Port (white)	Serve chilled sometimes with ice and slice of lemon/lime
Port (ruby)	Good ports served naturally. Lesser ports either by itself or with lemonade and ice
Sambucca	Coffee bean and set alight (For safety reasons this should be done at the table and the flame extinguished as soon as the oil from the bean is released into the drink)
Vermouths	With ice and slice of lemon/lime or sometimes with lemonade
Vodka	Tonic water or lemonade, ice and slice of lemon/lime; Orange cordial, ice and slice of orange; Lime cordial, ice and slice of lemon/lime; Tomato juice ice, slice of lemon and Worcestershire Sauce, sometimes with salt offered and also celery sticks
Whisk(e)y	Natural or with water (often still mineral water), with ice offered. Or with dry ginger or Canada Dry, or soda water and with ice offered
Wine	By the glass and sometimes, for white wine, with soda water or sparkling mineral water or lemonade, as Spritzer.
White rum	Natural with ice or with cola, ice and slice of lemon/lime

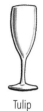 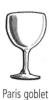

Cocktail   Saucer   Tulip   Flûte   Paris goblet   Elgin Liqueur

 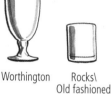 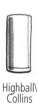

Worthington   Rocks\Old fashioned   Highball\Collins   Slim Jim   Sour   Brandy balloon   Port (Dock)

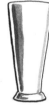 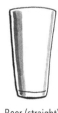

Lager/Pilsner   Beer (straight)   Beer (dimple)   Copita sherry   Elgin sherry

STORAGE OF WINE AND OTHER DRINKS

Key factors

- Good ventilation
- High levels of cleanliness
- Even temperatures of 13–15°C (55–59°F).
- Relative humidity of between 55–70 per cent be maintained.
- Strong draughts and unwanted odours should be avoided, so the cellar should be clean and well ventilated.
- Avoid intense lighting

Wine cellarage

Table wines should be stored on their sides in bins so that the wine remains in contact with the cork. This keeps the cork expanded and prevents air from entering the wine—a disaster which quickly turns wine to vinegar;

Special refrigerators or cooling cabinets can keep sparkling, white and rosé wines at serving temperature. These may be stationed in the dispense bar (a bar located between the cellar and the restaurant) to facilitate prompt service.

Storage of other drinks

Spirits, liqueurs, beers, squashes, juices and mineral waters are usually stored upright in their containers, as are fortified wines. If screw caps are used stand the bottles upright, if in cork, lay the bottles on their sides. Stopper caps and served caps are generally used for Sherries and most ports, which are also stored upright once opened. Vintage and crusted ports are stored horizontally but require time upright to allow sediment to settle at the bottom prior to decanting. Sherries rarely improve in bottle. Finos and Manzanillas and tawny ports are best consumed as soon as possible after purchase.

CIGARS

The main home of the cigar is Cuba and, to a lesser extent, Jamaica. Nowadays cigars are also made in a host of countries including the USA, Puerto Rico, the Philippines, Japan, the Dominican Republic, and the East Indies.

Sizes and measurements

There are 'classic' measurements for cigars, which many cigar makers attempt to follow. However the size of a cigar, when indicated by a name only, such as Corona or Robusto, is not an indication of a universal standard. Cigars are now categorized by length and Ring Gauge (also spelt Ring Guage), which is measured in multiples of 64ths of an inch.

Cigar Terms

Binder A single leaf of tobacco that is wound around the filler of the cigar to hold it together.

Bunch The term usually applied to the construction of the cigar when it consists of the binder tobacco wrapped around the filler leaves.

Curing The process of drying the moisture out of newly harvested tobaccos.

Filler The blended tobaccos, which form the inner core of the cigar. The filler is the most important part of the cigar as it is responsible for most of the flavour and smoking quality.

Long Filler Those fillers whose tobaccos run the entire length of the cigar. Long fillers are found in only the better cigars.

Shapes Cigars are made in a variety of shapes and sizes to suit the individual's preferences for taste and style. Many smokers select different shapes for different times of the day.

Wrapper The outer covering of the cigar is an important part of the cigar's flavour and smoking quality. The various shades of wrapper are: Claro (light, golden brown), Double Claro (result of picking the leaves before reaching maturity), Candela (light green), Colorado (reddish mid-brown), Maduro (darkest) and English Market Selection/Natural (lighter in colour than Maduro).

A cigar with a 52 Ring Gauge, for example, measures $^{52}/_{64}$ths of an inch in diameter. A Ring Gauge of 50 x 6 is $^{50}/_{64}$ths of an inch in diameter by 6 inches long. If the Ring Gauge is stated 6 x 50 it is still 6 inches long and $^{50}/_{64}$ths of an inch in diameter.

Storage

Cigars should be stored at a temperature of between 15°C and 18°C, (16.5°C is best), with a relative humidity of between 53 per cent and 57 per cent. Cedar wood boxes or cedar lined containers are ideal, as cedar, being porous, allows the cigar to breathe and the aroma of cedar blends well with that of a cigar. Using a humidor is also a good way of keeping cigars in condition. Sometimes when cigars are badly stored a greyish mildew or grey specks may appear on the wrapper. These can be wiped away quite easily with a soft brush. They are not harmful and neither are the yellow and green spots that are sometimes seen. The yellow spots occur through the sun drying rain drops on the tobacco leaves as they grow and the green indicates an over abundance of oil. Both demonstrate the authenticity and naturalness of the tobacco leaf.

Service

Cigar boxes should be opened carefully with a blunt instrument. To extract a cigar, press the rounded head and the cigar will tilt upwards for easy extraction. Customers should not be allowed to handle cigars before selection. In particular they should not be allowed to roll a cigar near their ear (sometimes called 'listening to the band'). This tells nothing at all about the cigar and simply damages it.

The band or identification tag should only be removed it the customer requests it. If it is to be removed it should be done carefully as moving it up and down can damage the cigar and even if peeled off gently, it can still rip the tobacco leaves.

When cigars are not pre-cut a V-shaped cigar cutter is required to cut the end (in a V), thereby facilitating maximum free draught and ease of smoking. Do not make a small hole with a match or cocktail stick, as this will leave a moist tar concentrate, which imparts a very bitter flavour as the end of the smoke is approached.

To light a cigar for a customer, use the broad flame of a long match, with a cedar wood spile or with a gas lighter, rotating the cigar to achieve even burning, and also periodically moving the cigar through the air to encourage burning.

Examples of cigars types and sizes			
Type	**Length inches**	**Length mm**	**Ring Gauge**
Torpedo and Pyramides	6–9	152–228	50–58
Belicoso	5–6	127–152	50–55
Robusto	4½–5	115–127	50–55
Hermoso	5	127	48
Double Corona	7½–8	190–203	47–52
Grand Corona and Montecrito A	9¼	235	47
Churchill	7	178	46–50
Corona Gorda	5½–6	140–152	46–48
Lonsdale Corona	6½	165	32
Corona Grande	6	152	42
Corona	5	127	40–43
Perla	4	102	40
Tres Petit	4½	115	40
Corona Culebras	5¾	145	39
Especial	7½	190	38
Long Panetela	7	117	35–39
Demi Tasse	4	102	30–39
Panetela	4½	114	26–33

PART 3: CUISINE, LAY-UPS AND ACCOMPANIMENTS

SAUCES

Although there appear to be a wide variety of sauces, they are mostly variations on the same base, or mother, sauces. These base sauces are:

- **Demi-glace**—Reduced basic brown meat sauce (espagnole).
- **Velouté**—Velvety white sauce using fish, meat, poultry or vegetable stock.
- **Béchamel**—Savoury white sauce made with milk.
- **Tomato**—Sauce made with fresh, tinned or puréed tomatoes.

For demi-glace, velouté, béchamel and tomato, a *roux* provides the basis for the sauces. There are three types: White (blanc), Blond (blond) and Brown (brun).

Other base sauces (emulsions) are:

- **Hollandaise**—Sauce made with melted butter, egg yolks, shallots, vinegar and peppercorns.
- **Mayonnaise**—Cold sauce made from egg yolks, oil, vinegar, salt, pepper and mustard.
- **Vinaigrette**—Cold sauce made from mixing oil and vinegar together with a selection of seasonings.

There are also the butter sauces (see page 118) and in addition to these sauces there is also Jus (gravy) and Jus lié (slightly thickened gravy).

Examples are:

- *Jus lié:* Stock thickened with cornflour or arrowroot.
- *Jus lié à l'Estragon:* As above with tarragon essence.
- *Jus lié Tomate:* Slightly thickened and flavoured with tomato.

Liaisons, starches, fecules and other thickeners and enrichers used in sauces include:

- **Blood:** For braised or roasted game, some poultry and rabbit dishes, sauces will have a mat appearance.
- **Bread:** In early times bread was an almost universal thickener.
- **Butter:** Mounting sauces with butter to enrich and give a gloss.
- **Coral:** A variety of shellfish coral can be used as final thickeners for sauces.
- **Cream:** Single and double cream, and whipped cream.
- **Egg yolks:** As fresh as possible.
- **Gelatin:** Commercial gelatine is almost colourless and transparent and is mixed with liquids and flavourings.
- **Giblets and foie gras:** Combine with half its weight in butter.
- **Starches:** Thickeners: e.g. roux, beurre manié, corn starch, arrowroot, potato starch, rice flour.
- **Yoghurt and fresh cheese:** (*fromage blanc*): Used to finish and thicken sauces.

Demi-glace—derivatives

Bordelaise: Chopped shallots, mignonette pepper, thyme, bay leaves, red wine, reduced, demi-glace, finished with butter.

Chasseur: Minced mushrooms tossed in butter, finely chopped shallots, white wine, reduced, demi-glace, finished with butter and chopped parsley.

Charcutiere: Robert sauce garnished with julienne of gherkins.

Chateaubriand: Sieved reduction of finely chopped shallots, thyme, bay leaves, mushroom pairings, white wine, finished with butter, tarragon and freshly chopped parsley.

Chevreuil: Sieved reduction of fried paysanne of onion and ham, butter and vinegar, port and red currant jelly.

Diable: Reduction of finely chopped shallots, pepper, white wine, and vinegar, finished with chopped parsley.

Diane: Poivrade sauce with cream added.

Duxelles: Onions and chopped shallots fried in butter, white wine, reduced, tomatoed demi-glace and dry duxelles, chopped parsley added.

Financière: Madeira sauce with truffle essence.

Grand Veneur: Poivrade sauce with venison flavour, mixed with red currant jelly and cream.

Lyonnaise: With sieved reduction of part fried onions, white wine and vinegar.

Madère: With butter, finely chopped shallots and Madeira, sieved and finished with butter.

Moscovite: Poivrade sauce, with infusion of juniper berries, garnished with grilled slices of almonds swollen in warm water, glass of Marsala.

Poivrade: Sieved with reduction of fried mirepoix of vegetables, parsley stalks, thyme, bay leaves, marinade and vinegar.

Réforme: One half poivrade sauce and one half demi-glace, garnished with short julienne of gherkins, white of eggs, mushrooms, truffles and tongue.

Robert: Finely chopped onions, butter, (no colour), white wine, vinegar, pepper, reduced, demi-glace, mustard to finish, sieved, monten au beurre.

Zingara: (a) Tomato demi-glace, garnished with mushrooms in julienne, truffles, ham, and tongue, cayenne pepper and Madeira; (b) chopped shallots reduced with vinegar, added to brown stock, brown crumbs, chopped parsley and lemon juice.

Velouté—derivitives

Allemande: Velouté cohered with yolk of eggs.

Aromates: Pale velouté mixed with an infusion of thyme, basil, marjoram, chives, chopped shallots, black peppercorns, garnish with chervil and blanched tarragon, lemon juice.

Aurores: Tomato fish velouté, butter.

Bonnefoy: Velouté and chopped tarragon.

Chaud froid: Velouté made with addition of aspic jelly.

Chivry: Chicken velouté, with infusion of chervil, parsley, tarragon, chives, pimpernel and white wine, strained and finished with Chivry butter.

Crème à l'Anglaise: Velouté with mushroom essence, flavoured with parsley and onion, cream.

Crevettes: Fish velouté with shrimp butter.

Curry: Dices of onion and apple lightly cooked in butter, add curry powder, moistened with coconut milk, velouté added, sieved and finish with cream.

Diplomate: Normande sauce with lobster butter, garnished with tiny dice of lobster and truffles.

Ecossaise: Normande sauce garnished with large brunoise of carrots, truffles and celery.

Estragon: Velouté with tarragon purée and chopped tarragon.

Homard: Diplomate sauce without garnish (see above).

Hongroise: Chopped onions partly fried in butter with paprika, moistened with white wine, faggot, reduce and mix with Suprême sauce (see below).

Ivoire: Suprême sauce with pale meat glaze.

Lagupière: Sauce bâtarde (white roux moistened with water, cohered with yolk of eggs, butter and creamed lemon juice and sieved) with fish glaze.

Nantua: Mirepoix of vegetables partly fried with crayfish butter, moisten with white wine and cognac, add fresh tomatoes and tomato purée, fish velouté, salt, cayenne pepper.

Normande: Fish velouté with mushroom essence and oyster juice, cohered with yolk of eggs and cream. Reduced and finished with butter and cream.

Persil: (For fish) Fish velouté, with an infusion of parsley, garnished with chopped parsley.

Riche: Same as Diplomate, which is Normande with lobster butter, small dice of lobster and truffle.

Régence: (For fish). Normande sauce, with reduction of white wine, mushroom parings, truffles, strained and finished with truffle essence.

Suprême: Chicken stock velouté, flavoured with mushrooms, finished with cream.

Victoria: Lobster sauce, velouté, chopped truffle.

Vin blanc: Fish velouté, thinned with fish stock, cohered with yolk of eggs, finished with butter.

Béchamel—derivatives

Cardinal: Béchamel with fish stock, truffles essence, lobster butter, cayenne pepper.

Crème: Béchamel sauce with cream.

Homard à l'Anglaise: Béchamel sauce with anchovy essence, garnished with dice of lobster, cayenne pepper.

Mornay: Béchamel sauce mixed with butter, grated gruyère and parmesan cheese.

Soubise: Béchamel sauce with cooked chopped onions seasoned and strained.

Shrimp: Béchamel sauce with shrimp dice and shrimp butter.

Tomato—derivatives

Chaud froid: Tomato sauce and aspic jelly.

Hussarde: Reduction of minced onions and shallots and white wine, and mixed with demi-glace flavoured with tomato, white stock, raw ham and garlic. Sieved and garnished with brunoise of ham, scraped horseradish and chopped parsley.

Tomato: Cold condiment. Tomato ketchup, hand made or proprietary.

Hollandaise—derivatives

Béarnaise: Hollandaise made with reduction of finely chopped shallots, mignonette pepper, tarragon, salt and vinegar. Finished with chopped tarragon and chervil to garnish the sauce.

Choron: As above blended with tomato purée.

Foyot: Bearnaise sauce with meat glaze added.

Maltaise: Hollandaise with zest and juice of blood oranges.

Mousseline ou Mousseuse: Hollandaise with stiffly whipped cream folded into it just before serving.

Moutarde: Hollandaise with mustard.

Noisette: Hollandaise sauce with nut brown cooked butter.

Rubens: Hollandaise made with reduction of white wine, fish stock and fine mirepoix, and finished with crayfish butter and anchovy pureé.

Sabayon: Made with reduction of fish stock, white wine, finely chopped shallots, egg yolks and butter.

Tyrolienne: Choron sauce with oil used instead of butter.

Valois: Same as foyot.

Mayonnaise—derivatives

Andalouse: Flavoured with tomato and dice of sweet pimento.

Gribiche: Mayonnaise made with hard yolk of eggs and mustard. Garnished with gherkin, capers, chervil, tarragon and julienne of hard boiled white of egg.

Marie Rose: Mayonnaise with addition of tomato ketchup (or juice) to taste, and Worcestershire sauce optional. (Used mainly for shellfish cocktails.)

Rémoulade: Mayonnaise sauce, mustard, garnished with capers, parsley, gherkins, chervil and tarragon, finished with anchovy essence.

Suédoise: Mayonnaise sauce with apple purée and scraped horseradish.

Tartare: Mayonnaise sauce, with lemon juice, chopped gerkins, capers and parsley.

Verte: Mayonnaise sauce with sieved purée of blanched herbs, spinach, watercress, parsley, chervil and tarragon.

Vincent: Half tartare sauce, half green sauce mixed together.

Vinaigrette—derivatives

Basic vinaigrette: For green salad: vinegar, salt, pepper, oil (some dry English mustard powder will act as an emulsifier).

Creamy vinaigrette: For salads: mustard, salt, pepper, vinegar, double cream, virgin olive oil, chopped chervil, chopped parsley.

Menthe: Mint sauce: finely chopped fresh mint, coarse salt, granulated sugar, vinegar, lemon juice.

Ravigote: Cold: wine vinegar, drained capers chopped, parsley, chopped chervil, finely chopped onion, salt, pepper, virgin olive oil.

Salsa verde: Garlic cloves chopped and crushed, parsley, basil leaves, virgin olive oil, capers, cornichons, mustard, wine vinegar, salt, pepper, breadcrumbs optional.

Note: other salad dressings are given on page 183.

Butter sauces—derivatives

Beurre blanc: Shallots peeled and finely chopped, white wine, white wine vinegar, double cream optional, butter, salt pepper. (Until the late 1960s known also as beurre Nantais).

Beurre Chivry: Parsley, shallots, tarragon, fresh pimpernel, and chives, blanched and pounded in a mortar with butter, and sieve.

Beurre citron: As beurre blanc, but with fresh lemon juice instead of white wine and vinegar.

Beurre de noisette: As beurre noisette but with purée of hazelnuts added.

Beurre fondu: Emulsified butter. Can be added to the likes of court bouillon, various stocks and cooking liquids. Also used for finishing last minute sauces rather than enriching with cold butter each time.

Beurre noir: Black butter. As for beurre noisette, but the lemon juice is replaced by reduced vinegar (used especially with skate wings).

Beurre noisette: Nut-brown butter. Melted and cooked butter until it breaks and colouring of the butter is stopped with lemon juice as it reaches a nut brown colour.

Beurre rouge: As beurre blanc but red wine instead of white wine.

HORS-D'OEUVRES AND OTHER APPETISERS

Hors-d'oeuvres

Traditionally hors-d'oeuvres are a selection of salads, fish and meats. The selection was served onto a cold fish plate and the cutlery was a fish knife and fork. The cutlery nowadays is more likely to be dictated by the type of food being served and its presentation.

Service can be a pre-plated selection or offered as a selection, in individual ravier dishes, from a tray, guéridon or from the traditional hors-d'oeuvre trolley. Oil and vinegar were also traditionally offered, but this has become less common because the foods are usually already well dressed. Brown bread and butter is also less often offered, thereby allowing the customer a choice of either butter or alternatives.

Common hors-d'oeuvre items include:

- **Salads:** Plain or compound. Examples of plain salads include fish and meat salads, cucumber salad, tomato salad, potato salad, beetroot salad, red cabbage and cauliflower. Compound salads include, for example, Russian (mixed vegetables in mayonnaise) Andalouse (celery, onions, peppers, tomatoes, rice and vinaigrette), Italienne (vegetable salad, cubes of salami, anchovy fillets and mayonnaise) and Parisienne (slices of crayfish, truffles, Russian salad and bound with mayonnaise and aspic). (See also page 180 for examples of other salads).

- **Canapés:** Slices of bread with the crusts removed, cut into a variety of shapes, then toasted or fried in oil or butter and garnished. Garnishes can include smoked salmon, foie gras, prawns, cheese, asparagus tips, tomato, egg, capers, gherkins, salami and other various meats.

- **Eggs:** These can be poached in aspic, hard-boiled, cut in two, garnished and stuffed with various fillings, which include the yolk.
- **Fish:** Items can include anchovies, herring (fresh or marinated) lobster, mackerel (marinated, smoked or fresh), smoked eel (filleted or sliced) and prawns (plain, in a cocktail sauce or in a mousse).
- **Meats:** Includes items such as foie gras, ham (raw, boiled or smoked) and salami of all sorts.

Other appetisers include:

- **Asparagus (Asperges):** Fresh asparagus can be eaten hot with, for example, melted butter or Hollandaise sauce or cold with vinaigrette or mayonnaise. It is useful to place an upturned fork under the right-hand side of the plate to tip the plate so that the sauce will form in a well at the bottom of the plate towards the left-hand side. Eating can be with a side knife and fork, with an asparagus holder or with the fingers. If with the fingers, then a finger bowl and a spare napkin should be offered.
- **Avocado:** Generally served in halves with a salad garnish on a fishplate. Can be served with vinaigrette (now more likely to be made with a wine vinegar), which is served separately, or with prawns in a cocktail sauce. There are also special dishes to hold half an avocado. Brown bread and butter is less common now. Alternative methods of presentation are also found, for example where the avocado is sliced and fanned out. A side knife and sweet fork are then laid.
- **Caesar Salad:** Salad of cos (or Romaine) lettuce, dressed with vinaigrette or other similar dressing, garlic, croûtons and grated (or shaved) Parmesan cheese. There are a number of variations to these ingredients. Cover is side knife and sweet fork. Sometimes this salad is served in a bowl.
- **Caviar:** Served with a caviar knife (broad blade knife) or side knife, on the right-hand side of the cover. Served onto a cold fish plate and accompaniments include blinnis (buck wheat pancakes) or hot breakfast toast, butter, segments of lemon, chopped shallots and

chopped egg yolk and egg white. Portion size is usually about 30g (1oz).

■ **Charcuterie:** This can include a selection of a range of meat (mainly pork) items including, Bayonne ham, salamis, smoked ham, Parma ham and also pâtés and terrines. Cutlery is a side knife and fork, or a joint knife and fork if taken as a main course. Accompaniments are peppermill and cayenne pepper, gherkins and sometimes onions. Occasionally a small portion of potato salad is offered. Bread is usually offered but brown bread and butter is now less common.

■ **Corn on the cob:** These are usually served with special holders which are like small swords or forks. Three wooden cocktail sticks in each end will also do the job, but avoid trying to use two sweet forks as it is possible to painfully catch teeth on the prongs. There are special dishes available, but a soup plate will do to provide a reservoir for the melted butter or Hollandaise sauce. A finger bowl and spare napkin might be advisable. A peppermill is offered.

■ **Fresh fruit:** Either served on a plate or in a bowl. Eaten with side knife and sweet fork if served on a plate and sweet spoon and fork if served in a bowl. Usually no accompaniment is offered although some people might like caster sugar. Both caster sugar and ground ginger are offered with melon if it is served by itself.

■ **Frogs legs:** Served on hot fish plate with lemon as accompaniment. Lay-up is side knife and sweet fork, and finger bowl and spare napkin.

■ **Fruit cocktails:** Usually served in a glass or some other form of bowl. These are eaten with a teaspoon and caster sugar is offered where there is grapefruit included in the cocktail.

■ **Fruit juices:** Usually served in a glass. Sometimes caster sugar is offered in which case a teaspoon should be given to stir in the sugar. For tomato juice, salt and Worcestershire sauce are offered, again a teaspoon should also be given to aid mixing in these accompaniments.

■ **Globe artichokes:** This vegetable is usually served whole as a starter. The edible portion of the leaves is 'sucked off' between the teeth after dipping them in a dressing (for example vinaigrette if served cold or melted butter or Hollandaise sauce if served hot). The leaves are held with the fingers. The heart is finally eaten with a side knife and sweet fork. A finger bowl and spare napkin are essential. There are special dishes for this vegetable, but a fish plate with a small bowl for the dressing will also do the job. In this case there would have to be a spare plate for the discarded leaves. Alternatively a joint plate may be used.

- **Lobster (homard froid) (cold):** Often served as a half with salad garnish and accompaniments are lemon and mayonnaise (or mayonnaise-based sauces). Lay up includes fish knife and fork, or side knife and fork, lobster pick and lobster cracker, debris plate and also finger bowl with additional napkin.

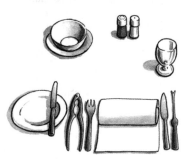

- **Melon:** Either served in halves, eaten with a sweet spoon, or in wedges or slices, eaten with a side knife and sweet fork. Traditional accompaniments are caster sugar and powdered ginger. Also often served with Parma ham eaten with side knife and sweet fork and there are no further accompaniments.

- **Mousses, terrines and pâtés:** Normally these are eaten using a side knife and sweet fork. Hot, unbuttered breakfast toast or another bread is offered. Butter may be offered and other accompaniments would be appropriate to the dish itself, e.g. lemon segments with fish mousses—although lemon is often offered with meat-based pâtés.

- **Niçoise Salad:** There are a number of versions of this salad. Generally it includes boiled potatoes, whole French beans, tomatoes, hard-boiled eggs (quartered or sliced) stoned black olives, flakes of tuna fish and anchovy fillets. This salad is usually made up and plated. Vinaigrette is often offered.

- **Other salads:** Salads can be made up and served plated or constituted at the guéridon. Dressings are various. Cutlery is usually related to the main ingredient i.e. fish knife and fork for fish-based salads, but a side knife and fork can be used for all. For further information on salads see pages 179–184.

- **Oysters (huîtres):** Cold oysters are usually served in one half of the shell on a bed of crushed ice in a soup plate. An oyster fork is usually offered but a small sweet fork can also be used. A finger bowl and an extra napkin could be offered as oysters are usually eaten by holding the shell in one hand and the fork in the other. Accompaniments include half a lemon and the oyster cruet 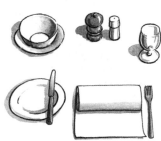 (cayenne pepper, pepper mill, chilli vinegar and Tabasco sauce). Traditionally brown bread and butter was also offered.

- **Potted shrimps:** A fish knife and fork or a side knife and sweet fork should be laid. Accompaniments include hot, unbuttered, breakfast toast (there is plenty of butter already in this dish), cayenne pepper, a peppermill and segments of lemon.

- **Seafood cocktails:** These are usually made up and served in glasses or bowls. A teaspoon and small fork are often laid for eating. Sometimes the cutlery is placed on the underplate and placed on the table with the dish. Accompaniments are lemon segment, peppermill, sometimes cayenne pepper and traditionally brown bread and butter, although this is less common now.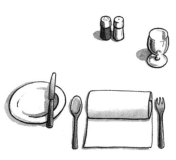

- **Smoked salmon (saumon fumé):** Usually eaten with a fish knife and fork or a side knife and sweet fork. Traditional accompaniments are half a lemon (which may be wrapped in muslin to prevent the juice squirting onto the customer when the lemon is squeezed), cayenne pepper, peppermill and brown bread and butter. Often nowadays a variety of unbuttered breads are offered with butter and alternatives served separately. Oil is sometimes offered and also chopped onions, capers and soured cream.

- **Other smoked fish:** As well as the accompaniments offered with smoked salmon, creamed horseradish has become a standard offering with all other smoked fish including trout, mackerel, cod, halibut and tuna.

- **Snails (escargots):** Snail tongs are place on the left and a snail fork on the right. The snails are served in an escargot dish, which has six or twelve indentations. French bread is offered for mopping up the sauce. Half a lemon may be given and a finger bowl and an extra napkin could be offered.

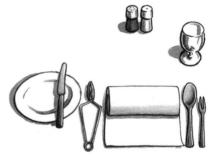

- **Whitebait (blanchailles):** Served on a fish plate and lay-up is a fish knife and fork, or side knife and sweet fork. Accompaniments are lemon, Cayenne pepper and peppermill being offered. Traditionally also served with brown bread and butter.

SOUPS

Soups may be divided into categories, including:

- *Bisque:* Thick soup prepared from crustaceans. Raw crustaceans impart the best flavour. A lot of the flavour also derives from the shells. Particularly good versions come from: lobster, crayfish, Dublin Bay prawns, prawns, shrimps, and crab.

■ *Bouillon:* Rich stock or broth.

■ *Brown:* For some time now these soups have been losing their popularity with customers. Brown soups are mainly British in origin. They are ideal lunchtime soups as they are usually robust and prepared from well flavoured stocks.

■ *Cold:* Ideal soups for the summer months where they can be welcome additions to lunchtime dinner and banqueting menus. These soups are best served ungarnished.

■ *Consommé:* Clarified bouillon. Can be made from poultry, beef, game, fish and vegetables. Also as *Consommé Double*—a concentrated consommé.

■ *Crème:* These soups are exemplified in their very smooth creamy texture and appearance. Classically cream soups obtained their creaminess from Béchamel as a 50 per cent volume in the soup. Today, they tend to be based on velouté and are finished with cream.

■ *Élixir:* Highly reduced consommé having a real extract of flavour and length on the palate. Can sometimes be seen with gold leaf.

■ *National:* National soups usually having special treatments.

■ *Petite Marmite:* Literally 'little pot' of clear, meat, poultry and/or vegetable soup served in a small *marmite* with lid.

■ *Pot au Feu:* Literally 'pot on the fire'. Virtually two dishes in one. Many regional variations exist. Usually with beef or poultry or both, but also with for example: salt pork and sausage. The meat that flavours the bouillon can be eaten apart or with the bouillon.

■ *Potages, soups and broths:* Most often based on distinctive, cut vegetables cooked in stock. These soups should not be over garnished. This style of soup is generally more suited to service at lunchtime as they tend to be robust. Examples include: Chicken and mutton broth, Scotch broth, Potage Cultivateur and Soupe à l'oignon gratinée.

■ *Purée:* Prepared from a base of fresh or dried vegetables. This also acts as their thickening agent. The process of puréeing or passing the soup is very important. The finished result should always be very smooth. The consistency of the soup is also very important—not too thin or thick. Purée based soups are usually consumed at lunchtime. The addition of a small amount of cream allows them to change their designation to a cream (crème) soup.

■ *Unclassified:* This section houses soups of a special nature not falling easily within any one of the other categories. Examples include: clam chowder, mussel soup, black cherry soup and potage Germiny.

■ *Velouté:* These soups need to have a velvety texture and sheen. They also tend to have a light delicate flavour. The soups are finished with a liaison of egg yolks and cream. Once the liaison is added the soups must not re-boil. Veloutés are based on the production of quality stock.

Service of soups

■ **Consommés:** Once drunk from the cup using handles and a spoon was provided to help with eating the garnish. This tradition continues with the use of a cup, but this is now presented at the table. The handles on some styles of cups have become merely representative ears. Although consommé is usually served hot it can also be served cold and jellied (en gelée).

■ **Veloutés, crèmes and purées:** Usually eaten from a soup plate with a soup spoon. It is however common now to see soup bowls of varying designs. Traditionally croutons were only offered with purées and cream of tomato soups but they are now commonly offered with a range of soups.

■ **Potages, broths and bisques:** These are also served generally in soup plates and eaten with a soup spoon, but again bowls of varying designs can also be used.

Examples of embellishments include:

Thickeners

■ **Flours:** Roux, beurre manié, potato flour (fécule), ground rice flour, arrowroot, tapioca flour.

- **Cream:** Single, double, whipped, crème manié (cream and butter).
- **Bread:** Crumbs, used extensively in Spanish and Tuscan soups.

Fortifiers
- **Wine:** Red/white.
- **Spirits:** Brandy, Madeira, sherry etc. vodka in consommé (as a pick me up).

Garnishes
- **Chiffonades:** Finely shredded vegetables, leaves of lettuce, spinach sorrel etc.
- **Pluches:** Small sprigs of parsley or chervil etc.
- **Vegetables:** Examples include: Brunoise, Julienne, Macedoine, Paysanne etc.
- **Savoury Pancakes:** As for crêpes with the addition of fines herbes, usually the crêpes are cut into a short julienne or small rounds whichever is more applicable.
- **Pastas:** Small pastas like vermicelli, stelline, ravioli.
- **Leaf:** Gold leaf or silver leaf.
- **Dumplings:** Various forms and flavours.
- **Meat Balls:** Various forms, sizes and flavours.
- **Royale:** Egg custard cut into various shapes having various flavourings
- **Profiteroles:** Unsweetened *pâte à chou* placed into a piping bag with a 3mm plain tube piped into pea-sized balls onto a greased baking sheet. These balls are egg washed and baked at 185°C until dry and crisp. They can then be stuffed with purées and served with for example consommé.

Accompaniments
- **Croûtes de Flûte:** Cut slices from a thin French loaf placed on a tray and lightly toasted on both sides
- **Croûtons:** Bread cut into ½cm cubes fried carefully in clarified butter till golden brown.

- **Sippets:** Tiny cubes of golden brown fried bread, or, thin slices of French bread dipped in flavoured oil and grilled.

- **Diablotins:** ½cm slices cut from a long thin French loaf, laid on a tray. Toasted on both sides until golden then sprinkled with Parmesan and Cheddar cheese.

- **Cheese straws:** Thin strips of egg-washed and parmesan-encrusted puff pastry, scented with cayenne pepper, twisted, baked in the oven. Cut into even sections.

- **Vegetable crisps:** Potato, carrot, swede, celeriac, parsnip, beetroot.

- **Caviar:** Sometimes served on toasts or on blinis pancakes.

- **Vegetable spaghetti:** Crisply fried vegetables which can be placed into the soup.

- **Wontons:** Meaning swallowing the cloud. Added to or served with the soup, various fillings.

- **Quenelles:** Made from many different forcemeats but force mousseline is best.

Examples of soups

Consommés

Ailerons: Garnished with chicken and rice.

Belle Gabrielle: Thickened with tapioca, garnished with rectangles of chicken, mousselline and crayfish tails.

Berchoux: Game consommé garnished with a royale (dice of set egg custard), blended with chestnut purée and quail essence, garnished also with julienne of truffles and mushrooms.

Bergère: Thickened with tapioca flour, asparagus tips, shredded poultry and pluches of chervil.

Boïeldieu: Chicken consommé thickened with tapioca garnished with three sorts of quenelles, foie gras, chicken and truffles.

Bretonne: Garnished with shredded leeks, celery, onions, mushrooms and pluches of chervil.

Brunoise: With vegetables cut into very small cubes.

Carmen: Made from the stock of tomato purée, sweet peppers. Garnish with rice and julienne of peppers, and chervil shreds.

Célestine: Thickened with tapioca flour, garnished with julienne of pancakes, mixed with chopped truffles or fines herbes.

Cheveaux d'Anges: Chicken consommé with small vermicelli. Parmesan cheese served separately.

Colbert: Poultry consommé. With printanière of vegetables and small poached eggs.

Crécy: Thickened with tapioca flour, garnished with Brunoise of carrots and pluches of chervil.

Croûte-au-pot: Petite marmite consommé garnished with a dice of vegetables. Serve croûtes apart.

Cultivateur: With very finely sliced vegetables and croûtons served separately.

Diane: Game consommé garnished with julienne of game, dice of truffles, and a glass of Madeira when served.

Double: Concentrated Consommé.

Ecossaise: Mutton broth garnished with dice of boiled mutton, pearl barley and large brunoise of vegetables.

Fermière: Poultry consommé with chopped vegetables and potatoes.

Floréal: Chicken consommé garnished with carrots, turnips, peas, asparagus heads, small quenelles with pistachio powder and chervil pluches.

Garibaldi: Chicken consommé garnished with perles du Japon (sago) and short strips of spaghetti.

Grenade: With tomato stock garnished with tomatoes and a tomato royale garnish.

Grimaldi: Made with tomato stock garnished with Julienne of celery.

Henri IV: A small casserole with the chicken cooked in it and croûtons served separately.

Julienne: Consommé garnished with julienne of carrots, leeks, turnips, cabbage, add peas, sorrel chiffonade and chervil pluches.

Léopold: Consommé with semolina. Garnished with chiffonade of lettuce, sorrel and chervil pluches.

Madrilène: Consommé with celery, pimento and tomato flavour. (Can be served cold). Garnish with tomato julienne, Pluches of sorrel and vermicelli (if served hot).

Monaco: Chicken consommé garnished with pea shaped truffles, carrots, turnips, and profiteroles.

Monte-Carlo: Chicken consommé garnished with roundels of carrots and turnips, stuffed pancakes and truffles.

Nelson: Fish consommé thickened with arrowroot, garnished with rice. Small bouchées filled with dice of lobster Américaine served separately.

Niçoise: Tomato consommé garnished with dice of tomatoes, French beans, potatoes and chervil pluches.

Parisienne: Consommé with leek flavour garnished with julienne of leek and potato.

Paysanne: Consommé with a Paysanne of vegetables. Serve croûtons separately.

Petite Marmite: Strong consommé of beef and chicken, garnished with carrot and turnip, leeks and cabbage. Julienne of celery, dice of beef and chicken. Serve in a special marmite. Serve small thin dry toasts separately.

Printanière: Consommé garnished with printanière of vegetables with peas and chervil pluches.

Profiteroles: Consommé garnished with tiny profiteroles.

Solange: Consommé garnished with pearl barley, squares of lettuce and julienne of cooked chicken.

Tosca: Chicken consommé thickened with tapioca flour flavoured with turtle herbs and Madeira. Garnished with tiny profiteroles and julienne of leeks.

Vermicelli: Consommé with vermicelli.

Vert pré: Consommé thickened with tapioca flour, garnished with asparagus heads, peas, French beans, lettuce and sorrel in chiffonade and chervil pluches.

Viveurs: Duck flavoured consommé with cayenne pepper, celery and beetroot juice. Garnish with julienne of celery, diablotins and paprika.

Xavier: Clear soup with chicken purée, royale garnish (dice of set egg custard), peas and chervil.

Veloutés, Crèmes and Purées

Agnès Sorel: A chicken velouté with mushrooms, garnished with julienne of mushrooms, white of chicken, tongue and a liaison with cream.

Ambassadeur: Purée of green peas garnished with rice, chiffonade of lettuce and sorrel, pluches of chervil, butter and cream.

Andalouse: Purée of tomato, rice and onions mixed with cream and garnished with boiled rice and julienne of capsicum (also *crème Andalouse*).

Argenteuil: Asparagus cream soup (also *velouté Argenteuil*).

Balvet: Pea purée:

Bisque de crevettes: Prawn velouté.

Bruxelloise: A purée of brussels sprouts.

Cambacères: One part pigeon velouté and one part crayfish bisque, garnished with pigeon quenelles stuffed with crayfish salpicon. Butter and cream is added.

Cardinal: A fish velouté with lobster cullis.

Céleri: Velouté with celery purée (also *crème de céleri*).

Chicorée: Velouté with endives, garnished with sippets, pluches of chervil, butter and cream (also *crème de chicorée*).

Choiseul: Lentil purée garnished with chiffonade of sorrel and rice. Liaison with cream and egg yolks.

Clamart: Purée of fresh peas. Garnished with croûtons.

Comtesse: (a) Asparagus velouté with chiffonade of sorrel, white asparagus heads and cream. (b) Haricots bean purée garnished with croûtons, pluches of chervil. Liaison of butter and cream.

Conti: Lentils purée garnished with a dice of fried bacon, Pluches of chervil, and butter.

Conti à la Brunoise: As above with a brunoise of vegetables.

Crécy: Carrots purée with rice. Butter and cream.

Crécy à l'Ancienne: As above with croûtons.

Crécy à la Briarde: Carrots and potato purée, garnished with croûtons, pluches of chervil and cream.

Cressonnière: Purée of potatoes and watercress, garnished with blanched watercress leaves. Cream or yolk of eggs.

Dubarry: Cauliflower velouté garnished with tiny florets of cauliflower, pluches of chervil. Cream. (also *Crème Dubarry*).

Ecrevises à la Joinville: Fish velouté with crayfish. Garnished with crayfish tails, julienne of truffles and mushrooms. Butter and cream. Fine Champagne when serving.

Egyptienne: Purée of yellow peas. Butter and cream.

Esaü: Lentils purée with rice. Butter and cream.

Faubonne: Purée of green peas, garnished with julienne of vegetables, pluches of chervil, butter and cream.

Flamande: Potato purée and brussels sprouts, cream or yolk of eggs.

Fontanges: Green peas purée garnished with pluches of chervil, chiffonade of sorrel. Butter and cream.

Freneuse: Turnip and potato purée. Cream and butter.

Garbure: A purée of vegetables. Butter and cream. Serve apart croûtons.

Gentilhomme: Purée of lentils with game stock. Garnished with a dice of ham. Croûtons. Butter and Madeira.

Germiny: Yolk of eggs blended with cream and butter moistened with boiling chicken consommé. Garnish with pluches of chervil. Serve cheese straws apart.

Homard à l'Indienne: As below with curry, garnished with rice.

Homard à la Cleveland: Velouté with cullis of American lobster garnished with a dice of lobster and a dice of tomatoes. Butter and brandy when about to serve.

Homard au Paprika. As for Cleveland with paprika and dice of pimentoes.

Indienne: Chicken velouté with coconut milk, flavoured with curry and garnished with rice. Cream.

Lavallière: ½ chicken velouté, ½ celery, ganish with royale, dice of celery, profiteroles served apart stuffed with chicken purée, cream and chervil.

Longchamps: Purée of fresh peas garnished with vermicelli, chiffonade of sorrel and pluches of chervil. Butter.

Longueville: As above substituting spaghetti for the vermicelli.

Maïs: Velouté of sweet corn garnished with grains of sweet corn. Cream.

Milanaise: Tomato chicken velouté garnished with dice of macaroni, julienne of white truffles, ham and mushrooms. Cream or egg liaison.

Montespan: Asparagus velouté garnished with tapioca, green peas, cream and eggs.

Montorgueil: Asparagus velouté garnished with a printanière of vegetables, chiffonade of sorrel, pluches of chervil. Cream.

Navarin: Purée of fresh green peas garnished with crayfish tails, peas, finely chopped parsley. Butter.

Palestine: Purée of Jerusalem artichokes Cream or egg yolks liaison.

Poireaux: Velouté with leeks. Liaison with cream or egg yolks. Serve croûtons separately.

Pois Frais: Purée of green peas garnished with peas, pluches of chervil. Butter and cream.

Pois Frais à la menthe: As above with the addition of blanched chopped mint.

Pompadour: Tomato purée garnished with sago and julienne of lettuces.

Portugaise: Purée of tomatoes. Garnished with rice. Butter.

Purée d'Oseille et Vermicelli à la crème: Chiffonade of sorrel cooked in butter and moistened with milk and consommé. Garnish with vermicelli. Cream and yolk of eggs.

Saint Germain: Purée of fresh peas, garnished with fresh peas. Butter and cream. Serve croûtons separately.

Solferino: Half parmentier, half cream of tomato, garnish with carrot balls and potato balls.

Xavier: Velvet soup with cream of rice, garnished with a dice of royale and chicken.

Soups or Potages

Agriculteur: A paysanne cut of vegetables cooked with lean bacon and served with croûtons.

Bonne Femme: Minced leeks and potatoes fried in butter, moistened with chicken consommé. Butter and cream. Serve with French bread.

Brésilienne: Carrots, turnips, leeks, celery, minced onions sweated in butter.

Cultivateur: Paysanne of vegetables tossed in butter with minced potatoes and salted pork. Moistened with white stock. Garnish with dice of pork.

Fermière: Paysanne of vegetables and cabbage julienne moistened with consommé. Serve slices of bread separately.

National Soups

Batwinia (Russian): Purée of spinach, sorrel, beetroot with white wine. Small ice cubes served separately. (serve very cold).

Bortsch (Polish): Duck flavoured consommé garnished with dice of beef and duck. Celery, fennel parsley roots, marjoram and peppercorns also feature as flavour enhancers. Scraped beetroot. Garnish with julienne of leeks, carrot, beetroot. Sour cream and beetroot juice. Small pies stuffed with duck forcemeat are served apart.

Bouillabaisse (French): Virtually a fish stew. Although a soup plate and soup spoon are used it is common for a knife and fork to also be given. Thin slices of French bread, dipped in oil and grilled are also offered (sippets).

Cerises (German): Broth made with Bordeaux wine or port, purée and juice of cherries cooked with lemon zest and cinnamon, garnish with stoned cherries and finger biscuits.

Cock a leekie (Scottish): Chicken and veal consommé garnished with julienne of leeks, prunes and chicken.

Hongrois (Hungarian): Dice of beef dusted with paprika tossed in butter and chopped onions. Flour is added and this is moistened with consommé. Garnish with dice of potatoes, Kümmel, crushed garlic. Croûtons.

Mille fanti (Italian): Consommé with a covering of bread crumbs, Parmesan cheese and beaten eggs.

Minestrone (Italian): Vegetable paysanne soup with pasta. Traditional accompaniments are grated Parmesan cheese and grilled flutes.

Moules Marniniere (French): (Mussels) Usually served in a soup plate or bowl on an underplate with brown bread and butter, or more commonly now various breads, and Cayenne pepper being offered. A fish knife and fork and sweet spoon are often laid for eating. A plate for the debris is often placed on the table together with a finger bowl and a spare napkin.

Mulligatawny (Indian): Chopped onions and apples fried in butter with curry flour and tomato purée, moistened with chicken consommé, add cream and garnish with a dice of chicken. Boiled rice

Petit Marmite (French): Beef and chicken flavoured soup garnished with turned root vegetables and dice of beef and chicken. Served in a special marmite pot, which resembles a small casserole. A sweet spoon is used to eat this soup, as it is easier to get this spoon into the pot. Accompaniments are grilled flutes, poached bone marrow and Parmesan cheese. Sometimes the bread and cheese are done as a croûte on top of the soup before serving at the table.

Soupe a l'oignon (French): French onion soup, often served in a consommé cup or soup bowl. Can be served with grilled flutes and parmesan cheese but is often topped with a slice of French bread gratinated with cheese.

Tortue Claire (English): Consommé of beef, chicken and turtle, flavoured with turtle herbs thickened with arrowroot. Embellish with Madeira wine.

EGGS

Egg dishes as separate courses have a chequered history. Omelettes have retained their popularity, but dishes such as eggs en cocotte only occasionally feature on menus.

Examples of methods of preparing eggs

- **Beaten egg poured in a thin trickle through a chinois into a boiling liquid, e.g., consommé** / *Oeufs filés*
- **Boiled egg served in its shell** / *Oeufs à la coque*
- **Eggs cooked in a fireproof dish** / *Oeufs sur le plat*
- **Eggs fried in moderately deep oil** / *Oeufs frit à la française*
- **Eggs presented in a cocotte dish** / *Oeufs en cocotte*
- **English fried eggs** / *Oeufs à la poêle*
- **Filled omelette** / *Omelette fourée*
- **Flat omelette** / *Omelette plate*
- **Fresh eggs newly laid** / *Oeufs frais*
- **Fried eggs** / *Oeufs frit*
- **Garnished omelette** / *Omelette garnie*
- **Hard boiled eggs** / *Oeufs dur*
- **Hen's egg, chicken's eggs** / *Oeufs de poule*
- **Moulded eggs** / *Oeufs moulé*
- **Newly laid eggs (today's)** / *Oeufs du jour*

- **Oval omelette** / *Omelette oval*
- **Plain omelette** / *Omelette nature*
- **Poached eggs** / *Oeufs poché*
- **Scrambled eggs** / *Oeufs brouillés*
- **Snow eggs** / *Oeufs à la neige*
- **Soft boiled eggs** / *Oeufs à coque*
- **Soft boiled eggs** / *Oeufs mollet*
- **Soft omelette (moist)** / *Omelette baveuse*
- **Stuffed eggs** / *Oeufs farci*

Eggs used can include

- **Plover egg** / *Oeuf de Pluviers*
- **Duck egg** / *Oeuf de Canard*
- **Quail egg** / *Oeuf de Cailles*
- **Goose egg** / *Oeuf de L'Oie*
- **Gull's egg (sea)** / *Oeuf de Mouette*
- **Hen or chicken egg** / *Oeuf de poule*
- **Turkey egg** / *Oeuf de Dinde*

Examples of dishes and their service

Oeuf sur le plat

The egg is cooked in the buttered oeuf sur-le-plat dish on the stove and sometimes finished in the oven having been placed in a shallow bain-marie, and then served to the customer in this dish on an underplate. A side knife and fork are used, but a spoon may be given depending on the garnishes. A sur-le-plat dish is a small round (usually white) earthenware or metal dish with two ears. Examples of dishes are:

Américaine: (1) Slice of grilled ham, break in the egg and when cooked surround with a thread of tomato sauce. (2) Garnish the bottom with scollops of lobster, break in the egg and cook, surround with a thread of Américaine sauce.

Bacon: Rashers of bacon, egg on top and cooked.

Bercy: Garnished with small grilled sausages and a thread of tomato sauce.

Egypienne: White of leeks and minced onions tossed in butter and cohered with cream sauce, cook the egg on top.

Estragon: Egg in the dish, with spoonful of thickened tarragon gravy, baked and decorated with tarragon leaves.

Florentine: Layered with blanched spinach leaves tossed in butter, egg on top and sprinkled with grated cheese, coated with mornay sauce and baked.

Gratin: Place mornay sauce on the bottom of the dish, and egg covered with mornay sauce and baked.

Lorraine: Garnish with rashers of grilled bacon and slices of gruyère cheese, with egg coated with thick cream and baked.

Lyonnaise: Garnish with onions tossed in butter, and garnished with lyonnaise sauce.

Meyerbeer: Egg fried off gently with grilled lamb's kidneys and coated with périgueux sauce.

Parmentier: Scooped out baked potatoes and half filled with purée, then egg and coated with cream and baked.

Parmesan: Sprinkled with freshly grated parmesan and baked.

Portugaise: Surround cooked egg with an even dice of tomatoes tossed in butter and tomato sauce.

Rothomago: Garnish with rashers of fried bacon or grilled ham, when the egg is cooked garnished with grilled chipolata sausages and add a thread of tomato sauce.

Savoyarde: Potatoes tossed raw in butter and sprinkled with grated cheese, egg on top and coated with thick cream and baked.

Victoria: Garnished with dice of lobster and truffles cohered with lobster sauce, and coated with lobster sauce.

Oeuf en cocotte

The egg is cooked in the cocotte dish, with various garnishes and also served in this dish to the customer. The dish is placed on an underplate and a teaspoon is used to eat the dish. A cocotte dish is a small round earthenware dish with straight sides. Examples of dishes are:

Bergère: Minced mushrooms and mutton, garnish with a thread of meat glaze.

Crème: Garnished with thread of hot thick cream when the egg is cooked.

Forestière: Diced fried bacon at bottom and sides with mushroom purée, garnished with chopped parsley when the egg is cooked.

Jus (au): Garnished with thread of reduced gravy.

Périgourdine: Foie gras slices at bottom, and garnished with thread of périgueux sauce.

Périgueux: Garnished with slice of truffle and a thread of périgueux sauce.

Portugaise: Tomato sauce at bottom, garnished with small dice of tomatoes tossed in butter with finely chopped shallots.

Reine: Minced chicken cohered with cream at bottom, garnished with thread of thick hot cream.

Saint Hubert: Interior coated with game purée, garnished with thread of poivrade sauce and a thin cross made from truffle.

Zingara: Garnish with thread of zingara sauce.

Omelettes

As an egg course an omelette is eaten with a joint fork and is served onto a hot fish plate. The joint fork is placed on the right hand side of the cover. Omelettes are often plated but may be served from a flat using two forks or two fish knives. The ends may also be trimmed as part of this service. They are at once simple and difficult to perfect, with tastes differing as to how they should be concluded. Some like the omelette *baveuse* (soft), with no colour and a perfect cigar shaped. Others prefer the egg well cooked and with colour, some like it just done and so on.

Garnishes have to be evenly cooked. Examples of dishes are:

Américaine: Filling of dice of tomatoes tossed in butter, the omelette is dished up on rashers of grilled bacon.

Andalouse: Filling of pimentos and tomatoes, surround the omelette with roundels of fried onions.

Angès Sorel: Stuffed with minced mushrooms tossed in butter and cohered with thin chicken purée, lay some roundels of tongue on top, surround with a thread of thickened gravy.

Arnold Bennet: Topped with flaked smoked haddock bound in fish velouté with egg yolk and cream, glazed and served flat.

Brillat-Savarin: Filled with dice of woodcock and truffles cohered with woodcock cullis, decorated with slices of truffle, surrounded with a good strong game gravy.

Champignons: Blended with minced mushrooms, decorate the finished omelette with slices of cooked mushrooms.

Crevettes: Split cooked omelette and filled with shrimp tails bound with shrimp sauce.

Espagnole: Blended with dice of tomatoes, julienne of sweet capsicums and minced onions cooked in butter. The omelette is served flat.

Fermière: Blended with dice of ham and chopped parsley. The omelette is served flat.

Fines-Herbes: Blended with finely chopped parsley, chives, tarragon leaves and chervil. The omelette is served folded.

Florentine: Blended with some blanched spinach leaves tossed in butter. The omelette is served folded.

Forestière: Filled with morels and cèpes, minced and tossed in butter cohered with meat glaze. Served with a cordon of thickened gravy.

Grand Mère: Blended with chopped parsley and a dice of fried bread. Served folded.

Hollandaise: Blended with thin scollops of smoked salmon tossed in butter. Serve a cordon of hollandaise sauce apart.

Jambon: Blended with dice of ham tossed in butter and the finished omelette is garnished with lozenges of ham.

Japonaise: Blended with finely chopped parsley and filled with Japanese artichokes blanched and tossed in butter and cream sauce.

Lard: Blended with a dice of bacon and served on rashers of fried bacon.

Limousine: Blended with a dice of potatoes and ham tossed in butter.

Lyonnaise: Blended with minced onions tossed in butter.

Maxim: Decorated with a row of crayfish tails and slices of truffle and then surrounded with border of frogs legs tossed in butter until they are well gilded and cooked to perfection.

Mexicaine: Blended with minced mushrooms tossed in butter and a julienne of sweet capsicums. The omelette is filled with a dice of tomatoes. Presented with a cordon of tomatoed demi-glace.

Nantua: Filled with crayfish tails cohered with nantua sauce, decorated with slices of truffles and crayfish tails. Presented with a cordon of nantua sauce.

Oseille: Blended with finely shredded sorrel tossed in butter. The omelette is served folded.

Parisienne: Blended with a fine dice of truffles and potatoes tossed in butter. The omelette is served flat.

Parmentier: Blended with some sauté potatoes. It is served flat.

Parmesan: Blended with freshly grated Parmesan cheese. The omelette is folded.

Paysanne: Blended with a dice of cooked bacon, potatoes tossed in butter, sorrel stewed in butter, and a pinch of chervil. The omelette is served flat.

Périgourd: Blended with a dice of truffles. The omelette is presented with a cordon of périgueux sauce.

Pointes d'Asperges: Mixed with heads of asparagus cooked in butter. The folded omelette is garnished with small faggots of asparagus heads.

Princesse: Blended with a dice of chicken and asparagus heads. The omelette is decorated with slices of truffles and small faggot of asparagus. It is presented with a cordon of suprême sauce.

Provençale: Filled with a dice of tomatoes tossed in butter with a little garlic. It is presented with a cordon of provençale sauce.

Reine: Filled with chicken purée. It is presented with a cordon of suprême sauce.

Savoyarde: Blended with potatoes tossed in butter. Slices of gruyère cheese are added. The omelette is served flat.

Suissesse: Blended with grated gruyère cheese. The omelette is sprinkled with grated gruyère cheese and glazed.

Oeufs Brouillés

Eggs in a pan with salt and pepper whisked and cooked over a bain-marie, finished with cream and butter to add richness. Examples of dishes are:

Archiduchesse: Combined with a dice of ham and mushrooms. Asparagus heads tossed in butter are dressed on top.

Cannelons: Puff pastry horns filled with scrambled eggs.

Champignons: Garnished with a dice of mushrooms.

Divette: Mixed with a dice of crayfish tails and asparagus heads. It is presented with a cordon of nantua sauce.

Espagnole: Presented in half tomatoes cooked in oil. Julienne of pimentoes on top.

Fines Herbes: Combined with chopped chives, chervil, tarragon and parsley.

Georgette: In baked potatoes, scooped, and filled with the eggs blended with crayfish, butter and crayfish tails.

Grand Mère: Combined with a dice of fried bread finished with chopped parsley.

Leuchtemberg: Combined with blanched chives. Serve caviar in the centre.

Magda: Mixed with chopped parsley, grated cheese and mustard, surrounded with croûtons.

Nantua: Combined with salpicon of crayfish and truffles, surrounded with slices of truffles. Presented with a cordon of nantua sauce.

Orloff: Cooked and served in cocottes garnished with crayfish tails with a slice of truffle on top.

Parmesan: Combined with parmesan cheese.

Pointes d'Asperges: Combined with asparagus heads. A bouquet of heads is presented on top of the eggs.

Sultane: Presented in potato croustades finished with pistachio butter.

Truffes: Combined with a dice of truffles. Decorate with large slices of truffles. A cordon of meat glaze is served.

Yvette: Garnished with asparagus heads and a dice of crayfish tails. The eggs are dressed in tartlets with a slice of truffle and a cordon of nantua sauce is served.

Oeufs Durs

Hard boiled eggs. Immersed in boiling water they are cooked for between 8–10 minutes, depending on how you wish to process them further. Examples of dishes are:

Aurore: Coated with tomatoed béchamel, topped with grated cheese and glazed

Chimay: Halved lengthways, and yolk passed through a sieve, mixed with dry duxelles and chopped parsley. Cream, salt and pepper added to the mix, and piped into the whites of eggs. Coated with Mornay sauce and glazed.

Granville: Cut into quarters and mixed with bordelaise sauce.

Hongroise: Cut into roundels, dressed in a dish with slices of tomatoes coated with paprika sauce containing sweated off minced onions.

Tripe (à la): Cut into roundels and mixed with onion sauce and chopped parsley.

Oeufs à Coque, Mollets, Moules et Poches

Boiled, soft boiled, moulded and poached. Examples are:

Africaine: Served on toasts, garnished with grilled ham, pilaw rice and dice of tomatoes.

Alsacienne: Placed on tartlets garnished with sauerkraut and a slice of ham.

Anglaise: On toast, sprinkled with Cheshire cheese and cayenne pepper, melted butter and gratinated.

Benedict: Poached eggs presented on ham on toasted English muffin, covered in hollandaise sauce, sometimes glazed.

Bombay: Served in timbales with curry sauce.

Cardinal: Served in tartlets garnished with a dice of lobster cohered with cardinal sauce.

Clamart: Served in tartlets, with green pea purée, coated with suprême sauce.

Coque (à la): Plunged into boiling water for 2–3 minutes.

Hollandaise: Served on croustades garnished with salmon purée and coated with Hollandaise sauce.

Indienne: Served of a bed of rice with curry and coated with curry sauce.

Lavallière: Poached egs, served in tartlets, garnish with sorrel purée with cream, coated with suprême sauce, decorated with asparagus heads.

Madras: Served in tartlets, garnished with rice. Coated with curry sauce.

Massenet: Applies to boiled, soft boiled, moulded and poached eggs, served on artichoke bottoms, garnished with small anna potato, egg is placed on potato and coated with cream sauce mixed with french bean purée.

Mollets: Eggs are plunged unto boiling water for 5–6 minutes, they are then cooled and shelled.

Moulés: Eggs cooked in buttered moulds, for 5–6 minutes in a bain-marie. Allowed to stand for a period then removed and unmoulded.

Pochés: Cooked in boiling water with a little vinegar and salt and poached for 2–5 minutes.

PASTA AND RICE DISHES

These dishes, which are also referred to as farinaceous dishes, include all pastas such as spaghetti, macaroni, nouilles, ravioli and also rice dishes such as pilaf, or risotto.

For spaghetti, a joint fork should be laid on the right-hand side of the cover and a sweet spoon on the left. For all other dishes a sweet spoon and fork are used. Grated parmesan cheese is normally offered with all these dishes. Sometimes the parmesan cheese is now shaved from the piece rather than being grated.

Examples of dishes are:

- **Cannelloni:** Small rolls of pasta filled with minced poultry or meat, but more frequently with minced meat and spinach, covered with a little tomato sauce and grated cheese and baked.

- **Lasagne:** Strips of pasta interlaced with minced meat, covered with a little tomato sauce and grated cheese and baked.

- **Gnocchi:** *Gnocchi Piémontaise:* made with potato, flour and eggs, rolled into small balls, poached then placed on an oven dish, covered with a tomato sauce, coated with cheese and lightly browned in the oven. *Gnocchi Parisienne:* made with choux paste and piped into small plugs, poached then covered with a béchamel sauce and grated cheese, they are baked in a slow oven so that they can both open out and become golden at the same time. *Gnocchi Romaine:* made with semolina, cut into various shapes, baked in the oven and served with a tomato sauce.

- **Pasta (macaroni, spaghetti, noodles, cornettes, penne etc.):** All these pasta are cooked in boiling salted water for between 12 and 16 minutes. Dishes include:

Arrabbiata: with chicken, spicy tomato sauce, basil and cheese.

Bolonaise: accompanied by a small amount of bolognaise sauce.

Carbonara : served with eggs, onion, olive oil, strips of bacon, cream and cheese.

Gratin: with butter to which a light béchamel sauce is added, covered with cheese and baked in the oven.

Millanaise: with butter and cheese, garnished with shredded ham, mushrooms and truffles and accompanied with a tomato sauce.

Napolitaine: with butter and cheese, mixed with a tomato sauce and a few small pieces of diced fresh tomato.

■ **Ravioli:** Small squares of pasta dough often filled with the same type of stuffing as is used for cannelloni. Poached in salted water, placed in an oven dish in alternating layers, first a layer of ravioli, then a layer of tomato and grated cheese, and so on, then covered with melted butter and baked or glazed in the oven.

■ **Rice: The types of rice dishes include:**

Pilaf: prepared long grain rice (white or brown) with onions and butter and cooked with a little bouillon so that it is quite dry and the grains separate easily.

Risotto: prepared short grain (white or brown) with onions, butter and a bouillon, but this time more copiously damped with the bouillon. When it is finished, it is bound with butter and grated parmesan.

À la grecque: pilaf rice, to which squares of dry sausage meat, peas and red peppers are added.

Millanaise: saffron rice risotto to which mushrooms and small squares of fresh tomato have been added.

FISH

Classic cuts of fish

- *Le Filet:* The fillet of fish removed from the bone.
- *La Paupiette:* Fillet of fish, flattened out, spread with a farce, then rolled.
- *Le Délice:* Trimmed neatly, folded fillet of fish.
- *Le Suprême:* Fillets of large fish, turbot, brill, halibut etc., cut on the slant.
- *La Darne:* A slice of round fish, cut on the bone.
- *Le Tronçon:* Slice of flat fish turbot, brill, halibut) cut on the bone.
- *Le Gougon:* Fillets of fish (usually sole) cut into strips.
- *Le Tranche:* A thick slice, portion or serving cut off the bone.

Preparation methods

- *Baked:* Many fish can be baked whole or in portions, either plain or with a savoury stuffing, often set on a bed of vegetables or can be baked with rock salt coating (eg as for Sea Bass)
- *Boiled:* Method used for whole fish such as salmon, turbot, trout and also for cuts from lager fish. Liquid used can be water, water and milk, milk, fish stock for white fish or court bouillion (aromatic stock) for oily fish
- *Deep fried:* Small or large fish cut into fillets, slices or goujons, dipped in milk and flour (à la Française) or flour, egg and breadcrumbs (pané—à l'Anglaise), and fried in very hot deep oil.
- *En papilotte:* Baked after enclosing fish, together with seasonings, in paper, or foil, envelope. Can be served from the envelope at the table.
- *Grilled:* Seasoned, dipped in oil and cooked on a very hot grill, or under a salamander, accompanied by a sauce or a composite butter.
- *Matelote:* The same method as for fish poached in white wine but the white wine is replaced by a good quality red wine.
- *Meunière:* Floured and shallow fried.

- ***Orly:*** Cut into fillets or slices, dipped in batter and deep-fried.
- ***Poached (hot):*** Cooked in an aromatic stock (court bouillon).
- ***Poached (cold):*** The same method as above but allowed to cool in the stock.
- ***Steamed:*** Alternative to poaching or boiling.
- ***Vin blanc:*** Poached in white wine. Covered with a white wine sauce to which is added the reduced stock from the cooking and with various garnishes.

Service of fish

Traditionally fish dishes were eaten with a fish knife and fork, but this practice is declining. For a fish course the usual lay-up is a fish plate and side knife and fork. For fish as a main course it is a joint plate with fish knife and fork or a joint knife and fork.

General accompaniments for fish are:

Hot fish dishes with a sauce	There are not usually accompaniments other than fleurons (small pastry items traditionally crescent shaped) served with poached fish dishes in sauces.
Hot fish dishes without sauces	Often have Hollandaise offered or another warm butter-based sauce served with them. Lemon may also be offered in various forms, e.g., half lemon wrapped in muslin, half lemon wedges, blanched lemon skinned and sliced etc.
Fried fish which has been crumbed (à l'Anglaise)	Often have tartare sauce, or other mayonnaise-based sauce, offered together with garnish of lemon and deep fried parsley.
Fried or grilled fish dishes not bread crumbed	Usually offered served with butter, if fried (*Meunière*), and plain if grilled, together with lemon. Sometimes sauces such as Hollandaise or tartare are offered. Grilled herring (*hareng grillée*) usually served with a mustard sauce.

Deep fried fish which has been dipped in batter (à l'Orly)	(Kitchen made) tomato sauce is sometimes offered together with lemon. Can also be served with cold mayonnaise based sauces or proprietary sauces together with vinegar if chips are also being served.
Cold poached fish dishes	Usually attractively garnished and served with mayonnaise or another mayonnaise-based sauce, such as Sauce Vert, together with lemon.
Hot poached fish dishes	Garnished with variety of sauces or served plain and generally accompanied with hollandaise sauce, mousseline or melted butter.

Categories of fish

Fresh Water Fish:

Bream	*la brème*	Lake trout	*la truite de lac*
Brown Trout	*la truite dorée*	Perch	*la perche*
Carp	*la carpe*	Pike	*le brochet*
Char	*la ombre chevalier*	Pike perch	*la zandre*
Chub	*le chevesne*	Salmon	*le saumon*
Dace	*le dard*	Salmon trout	*la truite saumonée*
Eel	*l'anguille*	Sturgeon	*l'esturgeon*
Farmed trout	*la truite fermière*	Tench	*la tanche*
Grayling	*la ombre de rivière*	Trout (river)	*la truite de rivière*
Gudgeon	*le goujon*		

Salt Water Fish:

Anchovy	*l'anchois*		Mullet	*la mulle*
Bass	*la perche*		Plaice	*la plie*
Brill	*la barbue*		Red Mullet	*le rouget (also known as goatfish)*
Cod	*le cabillaud*		Salt cod	*le cabillaud salé*
Conger	*le congre*		Sardine	*la sardine*
Dourad	*la dorade*		Skate	*la raie*
Flounder	*le flet*		Smelt	*l'éperlan*
Haddock	*l'aigrefin*		Sole; lemon sole	*la sole; la limande*
Hake	*le colin*		Tunny	*le thon*
Halibut	*le flétan*		Turbot	*le turbot*
Herring	*le hareng*		Whiting	*le merlan*
Mackerel	*le maquereau*			

Univalves are single shelled: Abalone and sea urchins are examples.

Bivalves have two shells joined by a hinge, such as clams, mussels, oysters, cockles and scallops.

Crustaceans are jointed exterior skeletons or shells such as lobsters, shrimps, prawns, crayfish, crawfish and crab.

Cephalopods The name translates as 'head-footed', and is a reflection of the fact that their tentacles and arms are attached directly to the head, examples are squid and octopus.

Examples of garnishing

For fish dishes the name of the fish being used is usually stated before the name of the dish as, for example, in Filets de sole Dugléré or Fillets of Sole Dugléré. Where the garnishing was originally associated with a particular type of fish, this is indicated in the list below. However, many garnishes are now also used for a variety of fish: for example the sole garnishes are often used for any white fish.

Admiral: Salmon, poached, coated with Nantua sauce and garnished with truffles.

Aïda: Turbot, filleted and poached. Dressed on spinach, season with salt and paprika, coated with Mornay sauce, sprinkled with cheese and breadcrumbs and glazed.

Aiglon: Sole, poached, dressed on mushroom purée, coated with white wine sauce mixed with soubise, cordon of meat glaze, served with fleurons.

Ambassadeur: Sole, poached, placed on a mushroom purée, covered with a white wine sauce and glazed.

Américain: Lobster or crawfish, cut into sections, seasoned, fried with chopped onions, garlic and shallots added. Flambéed with brandy. White wine, fish stock, chopped tomatoes, tomato purée and parsley added. Fish then coated with reduced sauce with pounded coral and butter added.

Américain: Sole, trout or turbot, filleted, poached, garnished with lobster collops and coated with Américaine sauce.

Argenteuil: Sole, poached, white wine sauce, white asparagus tips.

Belle meunière: Meunière, with addition of grilled mushroom, slice of peeled tomato and a flavoured and floured and shallow fried herring roe.

Bercy: Sole, poached in wine, shallots and chopped parsley.

Bleu: Trout, poached in water with salt and vinegar. Serve with plain boiled potatoes and parsley sprigs. Hollandaise sauce and melted butter is offered.

Bonne femme: Sole, poached, white wine sauce, mushrooms and glazed.

Bretonne: Meunière, with shrimps and cooked sliced mushrooms sprinkled over the fish.

Bréval: As for *bonne femme* with addition of tomato concassée.

Brillat-Savarin: Salmon, poached darnes, coated with sauce made from white wine, onions, celery, carrots, butter and cream and garnish with mushroom heads, olive shaped truffles and stuffed crayfish.

Caprice: Sole, bread-crumbed, grilled and garnished with floured and fried half banana, and Sauce Robert separately.

Cardinal: Lobster, cut in two, scalloped, coated with sauce Mornay and grilled.

Carême: Sole, poached, white wine sauce, oysters, mushrooms.

Carmen: Sole, poached, white wine sauce, tomatoes and tarragon.

Colbert: Whole sole opened along the back, bread-crumbed and fried. Part of bone then removed and bare area filled with maître d'hôtel butter.

Dieppoise: Sole, poached, white wine sauce, mussels and shrimps, cayenne pepper.

Doria: Meunière, garnished with cucumber.

Dugléré: Sole, poached, chopped shallots, white wine, tomato concassé, chopped parsley and cream. Garnished with chopped parsley.

Ecossaise: Salmon, poached darne, coated with white wine sauce with a brunoise of vegetables and truffles.

Florentine: Poached, on a bed of spinach, coated in Mornay sauce, glazed.

Grenobloise: Meunière, with capers, lemon and anchovies.

Hollandaise: Poached in stock with a separate Hollandaise sauce.

Hongroise: Poached, white sauce and paprika, crushed tomatoes and glazed.

Impérial: Salmon trout, skinned on one side, studded with truffles, braised in Champagne, garnish with prawns and poached herring roes, coated with white wine sauce and garnished with julienne of truffles.

Indienne: Sole, poached, curry sauce, pilaf rice served separately.

Kedgeree (Cadgery): Flaked poached fish (usually smoked haddock), mixed with rice pilaf, diced hard boiled eggs and with curry sauce.

Lagupière: Sole, poached fillets coated with white wine sauce, sprinkled with brunoise of truffles.

Marchand de Vin: As for *Bercy* but with red wine.

Marguery: Sole, as for *Bercy*, with addition of cooked prawns and 12 cooked mussels before coating with sauce and glazing.

Monte Carlo: Haddock, poached and garnished with slices of peeled tomatoes, or tomato concassé, poached egg and cream or cream sauce.

Mornay: Poached, coated with Mornay sauce and glazed.

Nantua: Sole, poached with a Nantua sauce.

Nelson: Turbot, poached, white wine sauce, glazed, garnished with noisette potatoes.

Newberg: Sole, poached, garnished with collops of lobster, coated with Newburg sauce and garnished with slices of lobster and truffles.

Newberg: Lobster, cut when raw, seasoned and sautéed in clarified butter and oil. Flambéed with brandy. Served with cream sauce made with residue in pan, Marsala, fish stock and cream.

Opéra: Sole, poached, white wine sauce, asparagus tips and truffles.

Princesse: Sole, poached, coated with white wine sauce blended with asparagus purée, garnished with croustades of Duchesse potatoes filled with asparagus heads and slices of truffles on top.

Riche: Sole, poached, Nantua sauce, prepared shrimps and truffles.

Richelieu: Sole, prepared as for Colbert but filled with maître d'hôtel butter and sliced truffles.

Saint-Germain: Bread-crumbed and grilled, served with separate Béarnaise sauce.

Sullivan: Sole, poached, coated with Mornay sauce, garnished with asparagus tips and truffles.

Thermidor: Lobster, in stock, cut into two parts; the flesh is taken out, mixed with cream sauce, re-stuffed in the shell and then baked.

Verdi: Whiting, filleted and poached, coated with Choron sauce and sprinkled with chopped truffles.

Véronique: Sole, poached in fish stock and Curaçao, cream and butter added, glazed and garnished with peeled, piped and poached muscat grapes.

Walewska: Sole, poached, garnished with lobster slices or tails and truffles, mornay sauce and glazed.

MEATS, POULTRY AND GAME

Beef

Roast beef (boeuf rôti) is served with roast gravy, horseradish sauce, French and English mustard and Yorkshire pudding(s). Other garnishes include:

Ambassadeur: Duchesse potatoes, artichoke hearts and mushrooms.

Bouquetière: Cauliflower, tomatoes, carrots, green beans and château potatoes.

Bruxelloise: chicory, brussels sprouts and château potatoes.

Clamart: Artichoke hearts, peas and château potatoes.

Dubarry: Cauliflower au gratin and parisienne potatoes.

Jardinière: Carrots, turnips, peas and cauliflower.

Printanière: New vegetables and new potatoes.

Romaine: Gnocchi romaine and spinach moulds.

Saint Germain: A purée of dried peas.

Sarde: Croquettes of rice, stuffed tomatoes and cucumbers *à la crème*.

Boiled Beef (boeuf bouilli)

Cooked in salted water, flavoured with vegetables and aromatic herbs. Accompaniments are turned root vegetables, natural cooking liquor, rock salt and gherkins. Boiled salt beef (silverside) is served with turned root vegetables, dumplings and the natural cooking liquor. Other presentations are:

Baveroise: Red cabbage, braised in red wine with bacon pieces.

Bruxelloise: Garnished with buttered brussels sprouts.

Flamande: With small braised carrots, cabbage and turnips.

Braised Beef

After first being marinated, the meat is braised in red wine. Examples of dishes are:

Bourguignonne: Garnished with small onions, salt bacon and mushrooms.

Bourgeoise: Garnished with small onions, salt bacon and carrots.

Other beef dishes

- ***Curbonnades:*** Slices cut mainly from the chuck, quickly shallow fried and then braised with onions and flavoured with vegetables and other flavours usually beer.

- ***Curry (Kari):*** General accompaniments are poppadums (crisp, highly seasoned pancakes either grilled or deep fried), Bombay Duck (dried fillet of a fish from the Indian Ocean) and mango chutney. A selection of sambals is also generally offered (see page 240).

- ***Estouffade:*** Small pieces of meat cut from the chuck, braised with bacon, onions, tomatoes and red wine, garnished with mushrooms and crushed tomatoes.

- ***Goulash:*** Cubes of meat braised with onions, paprika, bacon, and red wine. Often sliced potatoes are added to cook with the meat.

- ***Paupiettes:*** Flattened slices stuffed with minced pork, veal or fat bacon, then wrapped with a very thin slice of bacon fat and tied. These are then braised.

- ***Stroganoff:*** Sautéed strips of fillet, and served in sauce made with shallots, cream, parsley and white wine, accompanied by rice pilaf.

Steaks

Entrecôte (Sirloin)—entrecôte steaks are of varying thickness cut from the rib roast section and taking different names, depending on their size:

- ***Entrecôte minute:*** Thin cut or flattened to make very thin, then either pan-fried or grilled.

- ***Single Entrecôte:*** Regular size steak cut for one person and is generally grilled.

- ■ *Double Entrecôte:* Steak cut for two persons which is generally grilled or pan-fried.

- ■ *Entrecôte château:* Large steak in a single piece for 3–5 persons, grilled or pan-fried, but can also be roasted. Carved at an angle for service.

- ■ *Porterhouse Steak:* Thick cut across the sirloin including the bone.

- ■ *T bone:* Thick cut across both the fillet and the sirloin, including the bone.

Other steaks are fillet and rump steak. Châteaubriand is a large fillet steak (usually for two persons), which is grilled or roasted and carved at an angle for service.

Steaks are often served with various mustards and sometimes proprietary sauces as accompaniments and also with sauces such as béarnaise, choron, bordelaise, marchand de vin, maître d' hôtel, etc. Other garnishes include:

Américaine: Grilled with a fried egg placed on top and a cordon of tomato sauce around.

Forestière: With ordinary mushrooms or cèpes or morel mushrooms, dice of bacon and Parmentier potatoes.

Hongroise: Coated with hongroise sauce, garnished with bacon and potatoes à l'Anglaise.

Lyonnaise: Sautéed with sliced onions and coated with a demi-glace sauce.

Marchand de vin: Coated with red wine demi-glace (and in the past with chopped poached bone marrow).

Tyrolienne: Fried onion rings in batter and crushed tomatoes.

Vert-Pré: Grilled tomato, mushrooms, pommes paille (straw potatoes) and watercress. Maître d'hôtel butter served apart.

Veal (*veau*)

Blanquette

This form of cooking can be used for almost all white meats, but its main application is for veal. Small cubes of meat are cooked with vegetables and aromatic flavouring. The basic juices are used to make a white sauce and this is then coated over the meat. The blanquette is generally accompanied by a small garnishing known as *ancienne* and this comprises small onions and quartered mushrooms.

Escalopes, Médaillons and Grenadins

Escalopes are slices cut from the 'noix' of the veal which is roughly the same as the topside of the leg in a beef cut.

Médaillons: are medallion shaped pieces of veal, cut from the fillet and cushion of veal.

Grenadins: are noisettes with pieces of fat bacon inserted into them.

Garnishes include:

À la crème: Sautéed and coated with sauce made in the pan with cream, and lemon juice.

Bordelaise: With cèpes and bordelaise sauce added.

Chasseur: Coated with chasseur sauce.

Holstein: Panéed and sautéed and garnish with a fried egg, and a criss-cross of anchovy, served with a cordon of beurre noisette.

Milanaise: Panéed and with criss-cross made with the back of a knife on the presentation side and sautéed. Sauce made in the pan with julienne of tongue, ham, mushrooms, and truffles, sweat in butter and deglaze with Madeira and added to spaghetti cohered with tomato sauce, grated cheese and butter. The escalopes are presented with the spaghetti either at the side or with the escalopes on top of the spaghetti.

Viennoise: (1) Panéed with blanched peeled slice of lemon on each escalope and a stuffed olive surrounded by an anchovy fillet on top. Decorate a corner of the presentation dish with a 'v' shape of small capers, build out the 'v' shape with finely grated yolk of egg, chopped parsley and grated white of egg, hold this in place with thin anchovy slices. Cordon of demi-glace and coated with beurre noisette. (2) (Schnitzel) panéed and pan-fried. Serve with lemon and parsley.

157

Zingara: Panéed and cooked in oil, zingara sauce and garnish.

Veal cutlets and steaks

Cutlets are fairly thick strips cut from the flank, whereas steaks are cut from the saddle. These pieces of meat are normally fried in butter or are grilled. Garnishes include:

À la crème: Pan-fried and coated with cream sauce.

Chasseur: Pan-fried, coated with chasseur sauce.

Fermière: Casserole with paysanne of vegetables.

Maraîchère: Pan-fried serve with green beans and sautéed salsify, château potatoes and thickened gravy.

Milanaise: As per escalopes of veal.

Paprika: Dusted with flour and paprika, pan-fried and coated with sauce made in the pan by adding cream.

Pojarski: Shaped cutlets, made with veal forcemeat mixture, to form a cutlet with bone added, then panéed and sautéed.

Veal Fillet

Fillet of veal is normally used for noix de veau. Sliced into very thin strips, the meat is quickly fried in butter. Served with a cream or white wine sauce, or with curry, madeira sauce etc.

Mutton and lamb

Roast lamb (agneau rôti) is accompanied by roast gravy and mint sauce and also today more commonly, redcurrant jelly. Roast mutton (mouton rôti) was traditionally accompanied by redcurrant jelly and sometimes white onion sauce (soubise). Boiled mutton (mouton bouilli) is accompanied by caper sauce.

Irish Stew

This stew, made from scrag end, is often served in a hot soup plate on a cold joint plate (underplate) and a sweet spoon is offered together with the joint knife and fork. Accompaniments are Worcestershire sauce and pickled red cabbage.

Leg and Shoulder

Leg and shoulder is normally roasted but it can be boiled. Garnishes include:

À l'Anglaise: Boiled, with carrots, turnips, cabbage and potatoes.

Boulangère: Roasted, with sliced potatoes and chopped onions cooked in bouillon or consommé.

Bretonne: Roasted, with haricot beans and château potatoes.

Menthe: Roasted or boiled, with mint sauce.

Printanière: Roasted, with carrots, turnips, peas, French beans and new potatoes.

Tourangelle: Roasted, with green beans mixed with broad beans.

Cutlets and Chops

Presentations include:

Bretonne: Pan-fried, and garnished with broad beans.

Champvalon: Pan-fried and then baked covered with onions and sliced potatoes, and with meat stock or consommé. Garnished with parsley.

Dubeley: Grilled, garnished with grilled mushrooms.

Maréchale: Garnished with asparagus tips and slices of truffles.

Parisienne: Grilled, with asparagus tips and parisienne potatoes.

Pompadour: Grilled, with asparagus tips and artichoke hearts.

Pork

Roast pork (porc rôti) is served with roast gravy, sage and onion stuffing and apple sauce.

Cutlets and Chops

Presentations include:

Bruxelloise: Pan-fried, with Brussels sprouts in butter.

Charcutière: Pan-fried, coated with charcutière sauce.

Flamande: Pan-fried, cooked with sliced apples.

Millanaise: As per escalopes of veal.

Normande: Pan-fried, served with apple sauce.

Robert: Grilled, served with robert sauce.

Ham

The ham can be, depending on circumstances, boiled or braised. Boiled ham (jambon bouilli) can be accompanied by parsley sauce or white onion sauce (soubise). Other garnishes include:

Alsacienne: Sauerkraut and buttered potatoes.

Bourguignonne: Braised in red wine, with mushrooms and small onions.

Kidneys and liver (rognons et foie)

Kidneys (calf, ox and lamb)

Américaine: Grilled with tomatoes and grilled bacon.

Bordelaise: Sautéed, with red wine, mushrooms, pieces of bacon and onions in demi-glace.

Brochette: On a skewer with diced cèpes mushrooms.

Madère: Pan-fried and mixed with madeira sauce.

Orientale: Cut in pieces, pan-fried and served with pilaf rice and tomato sauce.

Turbigo: Cut, sautéed and garnished with grilled chipolatas and sautéed mushrooms, covered with sauce of cooking liquor, white wine and tomato demi-glace served into heart-shaped crôutons.

Vert-Pré: Grilled, with maître d'hotel butter, tomato, mushrooms, watercress and pommes paille.

Liver (lamb, ox or calf)

À l'Anglaise: Sliced, grilled and covered with slices of grilled bacon.

Bercy: Sliced, grilled, with bercy butter.

Lyonnaise: Sliced, sautéed, garnished with fried diced bacon.

Sauté: Finely chopped and quickly fried, mixed with demi-glace sauce and with white wine, madeira etc.

Mixed grill and other grills

These dishes are generally garnished 'vert pré'—watercress, grilled tomato, grilled or sautéed mushrooms and pommes paille (deep fried straw potatoes) and a sauce boat of beurre maître d'hotel (parsley butter) is served apart. Various mustards and sometimes proprietary sauces act as accompaniments (see also Steaks page 155).

Noisettes, tournedos, filets mignons (lamb, beef and mutton)

These are slices cut from the fillet of beef, lamb or mutton and can be either grilled or pan-fried. They are often accompanied with various sauces such as béarnaise, choron, foyot, bordelaise, maître d' hôtel, bercy etc. In addition to the presentation identified about, other general presentation include:

Alexandra: Garnished with slices of truffles and artichoke bottoms.

Baron Brisse: Sauteed, slice of tomato on top of each, garnished with soufflé potatoes and artichoke bottoms filled with tiny truffle balls, demi-glace sauce.

Bruxelloise: Coated with madeira sauce, garnish with brussels sprouts, braised chicory and château potatoes.

Châtelaine: Garnish with noisette potatoes and artichoke bottoms.

Choron: Pan-fried, garnished with artichoke bottoms filled with fresh peas, and garnished with noisette potatoes.

Clamart: Coated with madeira sauce, garnish with artichoke bottoms filled with green peas.

Dauphine: Coated with madeira sauce, garnish with dauphine potatoes.

Dubarry: Coated with madeira sauce, surround with small cauliflowers coated with mornay sauce and glazed.

Dugléré: Set on a croûton, garnished with whole tomatoes peeled and cooked, chicory and mushrooms, coated with demi-glace.

Fleuriste: Coated with demi-glace, garnished with halves of tomatoes filled with jardinière.

Forestière: Set on a croûton, garnish with morels, bacon and parmentière potatoes.

Helder: Thread of béarnaise sauce around the edge of the tournedos and a dice of tomatoes in the centre. Garnished with parisienne potatoes, Coated with veal gravy and madeira sauce.

Lakmé: Topped with grilled mushrooms dressed on tartlets filled with broad bean purée, serve with thickened gravy.

Massenet: Pan-fried, garnished with artichoke bottoms filled with marrow, french beans and anna potatoes.

Mirabeau: Anchovy fillets in a criss cross across the steak with sliced stuffed olives filling in the hollows in the anchovy crosses and tarragon leaves.

Montpensier: Garnished with artichoke bottoms filled with asparagus heads, cohered with butter, coated with madeira sauce and truffles julienne.

Nancy: As for Rossini without the truffle.

Périgourdine: As for Rossini without the foie gras.

Piémontaise: Garnished with tartlets filled with risotto à la piémontaise. Coated with madeira sauce.

Portugaise: Dice of cooked tomatoes on top and coated with tomatoed madeira sauce.

Princesse: Garnished with bouquets of asparagus heads and a slice of truffle. Coated with white wine demi-glace.

Provençale: Provençal sauce and garnished with olives, mushrooms and served with croquette potatoes.

Saint-Germain: Purée of dried green peas and coated with béarnaise sauce.

Valenciennes: Presented on pilaw rice containing a dice of red pimentoes. Coated with white wine demi-glace.

Valois: Presented on *Anna* potato crouton, coated with white wine demi-glace, and garnished with sliced artichoke bottoms.

Rossini: Set on a croûton with foie gras collop on top of the fillet and with a slice of truffle in the centre, coated with madeira sauce.

Verdi: Pan-fried, set on a foie-gras crouton and coated with sauce soubise (onion sauce), glazed, and garnished with croustades made with pommes duchesse filled with tiny carrot balls, alternated with braised lettuces and a cordon of madeira demi-glace.

Poultry (*volaille*)

The term is applied to all domestic birds. Poultry is classified into two groups, the white fleshed and the dark fleshed varieties. In the first group are the birds that go under the names: chicken, fattened chicken, capon, pullet, grain chicken, spring chicken, and turkey. In the second group are: ducks, geese, and guinea fowl.

Dishes and accompaniments

Roasted:

- **Roast chicken (poulet rôti):** Accompaniments are bread sauce, roast gravy and parsley and thyme stuffing, sage and onion stuffing. Watercress and game chips (crisps) are also served.

- **Roast duck (caneton rôti):** Sage and onion stuffing, apple sauce and roast gravy. Watercress and game chips (crisps) are also served.

- **Wild duck (caneton sauvage):** Roast gravy and traditionally an orange salad with an acidulated cream dressing is offered as a side dish. Watercress and pommes gaufrettes (deep fried lattice work thin slices of potato) are also offered.

- **Roast goose (oie rôti):** Sage and onion stuffing, apple sauce and roast gravy. Watercress and game chips (crisps) are also served.

- **Roast turkey (dinde rôti):** Cranberry sauce, chestnut stuffing, chipolata sausages, game chips (crisps) watercress and roast gravy are the usual accompaniments.

Other presentations for poultry include:

Ancienne: Pan-fried, small onions, mushrooms and croûtons.

Angès Sorel: Poach supreme, dressed on tartlets lined with mushrooms and forcemeat, coated with suprême sauce and decorated with tongue and truffles, cordon of pale meat glaze.

Argenteuil: Braised and garnished with asparagus tips.

Beaulieu: Sautéed, coated with pan-made sauce with addition of white wine and veal stock, garnished with artichoke bottoms in quarters, tomato concassé and stoned black olives. Served with cocotte potatoes.

Belle Gabrielle: Sautéed without colour, coated with pan-made sauce with addition of cream and suprême sauce, sprinkled with chopped truffles, and heart shaped croutons.

Bergère: Sautéed without colour, served with pan-made sauce with additions of madeira, veal stock, cream, and garnished with sauté mushrooms, and thin chipped potatoes.

Bonne Femme: Sautéed, coated with pan-made sauce with addition of white wine, thickened gravy, garnish with dice of bacon, small onions, and cocotte potatoes.

Bordelaise: Sautéed, white wine, demi-glace, chopped shallots, garnish with artichoke bottoms in quarters, roundels of fried onions and sauté potatoes.

Bourgignonne: Sautéed, coated with pan-made sauce with addition of red wine, demi-glace, chopped garlic, garnish with glazed onions, dice of bacon and mushrooms, and finished with finely chopped parsley.

Chasseur: Sautéed, coated with pan-made sauce with addition of white wine, brandy, tomatoed demi-glace, sliced mushrooms tossed in butter with chopped shallots, finished with finely chopped parsley.

Chivry: Boiled, served with a suprême sauce, garnish with mixed diced vegetables.

Estragon: Sautéed, coated with pan-made sauce with addition of white wine, chopped shallots and chopped tarragon, thickened gravy and cream, and decorate with tarragon.

Fermière: Sautéed, thickened gravy, cooking completed in a cocotte dish, garnish with carrots, turnips, lettuce and peas.

Financière: Casserole, garnish with mushrooms, truffles, olives and Financière sauce.

Forestière: Casserole, garnished with morel or cèpes mushrooms and parmentière potatoes.

Hongroise: Sautéed coated with pan-made sauce with addition of paprika and chopped onion, cream, hongroise sauce and tomato concassé, and bordered with pilaf rice.

Indienne: Curried.

Ivoire: Poached and served with suprême sauce.

Marengo: Sautéed, coated with pan-made sauce with addition of white wine, tomato concassé, tomatoed demi-glace, chopped garlic, mushroom heads, slices of truffles, garnished with crayfish, and garnished with french fried eggs, croûtons and chopped parsley.

Monselet: Sautéed, coated with pan-made sauce with addition of, sherry, demi-glace, artickoke bottoms in quarters, slices of truffles.

Morilles: Sautéed, coated with pan-made sauce with addition of morels, brandy, meat glaze, and cooking liquor from the morels, finish monten au beurre.

Paysanne: Sautéed, coated with pan-made sauce with addition of white wine and paysanne of vegetables.

Périgord: Sautéed with truffles, coated with madeira, and buttered demi-glace sauce.

Portugaise: Sautéed, coated with pan-made sauce with addition of chopped onions, white wine, dice of tomatoes, sliced mushrooms, a little chopped garlic, surrounded with stuffed tomatoes.

Princesse: Poached, suprême sauce and asparagus heads added.

Renaissance: Boiled, with artichoke hearts, asparagus tips and a suprême sauce.

Other presentations for duck, duckling and goose include:

Bigarade: Casseroled, garnished with orange quarters and orange sauce.

Orange: Braised, with a demi-glace sauce made with orange juice and garnished with orange fillets.

Montmorency: Pot-roasted with herbs, and garnished with stoned (Montmorency) cherries poached in Bordeaux wine.

Guinea Fowl

All the cooking methods described for pheasants and partridges (see page 167) and the garnishes that normally accompany chicken (see above) can be applied to this bird.

Pigeon

Allemande: Cooked in a casserole with a pepper cream sauce.

Bonne femme: Casseroled with small onions and mushrooms.

Crapoudine: Flattened, partially boned and formed into a toad shape, dipped, grilled and served with a separate sauce diable.

Petits pois: Casseroled, garnished with peas à la française.

Pigeon pie: Half roasted then placed in a soufflé dish, covered with pieces of grilled bacon, parisienne potatoes, mushrooms, hard boiled eggs, and stoned olives, then encased in puff pastry.

Furred game

Hare (lièvre)

À la crème: Roasted, with cream sauce.

Forestière: Roasted, with mushrooms, glazed chestnuts and a poivrade sauce.

Grand-Veneur: Roasted in a casserole, with a grand-veneur sauce, chestnut purée and redcurrant jelly.

Civet de lièvre: Jugged Hare, braised and garnished with button onions, mushrooms, bacon, heart shaped croutons with the tips dipped in demi-glace then finely chopped parsley, forcemeat balls and redcurrant jelly.

Saint Hubert: Rabbit or hare, larded and marinated. Cooked in a casserole, served coated with poivrade sauce, surrounded with grilled mushrooms garnished with game purée.

Venison (venaison)

When roasted, served with roast gravy and Cumberland sauce and also/or redcurrant jelly. Other garnishes include:

Cutlets and noisettes
Badoise: Pan-fried with s pepper sauce mixed with cream and cherry juice.

Diane: Pan-fried, with sliced mushrooms and bacon, and a chasseur sauce.

Venaison: Sautéed, coated with a poivrade sauce to which redcurrant jelly has been added, and chestnut purée.

Saddle
Badoise: Roast with stoned cherries and poivrade sauce.

Cumberland: Roast, with chestnut purée and cumberland sauce.

Grand-Veneur: Spiked, marinated and roasted, with chestnut purée and grand-veneur sauce.

Metternich: Roast, with chestnuts, red cabbage, apples filled with redcurrant jelly and grand-veneur sauce.

Feathered game

When roasted, the accompaniments for all feathered game, including for instance partridge (perdreau), grouse ([red] lagopède, [male] rouge d'Ecosse) and pheasant (faisan) are fried breadcrumbs, hot liver pâté spread on a croûte on which the meat sits, bread sauce and pommes gaufrettes, watercress and roast gravy are also served. Other presentations include:

Partridge, Pheasant and Wood grouse
Bohémienne: As for chartreuse, with sauerkraut.

Chartreuse: Pieces of roast pheasant covered with braised savoy cabbage, decorated with slices of carrot, lean bacon, and sausage, around a pheasant base.

Salmis: Roasted, cut up and cooked in a salmis sauce.

Smitane: Sautéed, coated with smitane sauce.

Quail

Broche: Roasted on a skewer (*en brochet*).

Périgourdine: In a casserole, with truffles and mushrooms.

Saint Hubert: Cooked in a cocotte with a truffle inside the bird. Sauce made with cooking liquor, madeira and game stock, previously garnished with cocks, combs and truffles.

Souvaroff: As for the woodcock.

Vigneronne: roasted in a casserole and garnished with muscat grapes in a madeira and curaçao sauce.

Woodcock and Snipe

Crème: Sautéed, served with a cream sauce.

Financière: Sautéed, garnished with a financière ragoût and a madeira sauce.

Grilled: Split down the middle, dipped, grilled and served with a diable sauce.

Hongroise: As for crème with the addition of paprika.

Souvaroff: Stuffed with foie gras and truffles, cooked in a casserole which is sealed with pastry, around the edge of the lid.

NOTES ON CARVING

The carving of meats is a skill that is developed only through practice. The two most important things in carving are a sharp knife (blunt ones cause accidents) and confidence. Some general points to consider are:

- Meat is generally carved across the grain.
- Always use a very sharp knife. For most joints use a knife with a blade 25–30cm (10–12 in) long and about 2.5cm (1 in) wide; for poultry or

game it is best to use a knife with a blade 20cm (8 in) long; for ham a long, flexible carving knife is used often called a ham knife. Serrated knives do not always cut better than plain bladed knives, which give a cleaner cut.

- When carving or jointing, the meat should be held firmly, usually with a carving fork, in order to avoid accidents.
- Carve on a board (either wooden or plastic). Avoid carving on plates or metal. Apart from the damage this can cause, especially to silver, in the case of metal, small splinters of metal can become attached to the meat slices.

Methods of carving:

- Chicken—medium-sized birds are often dissected into eight pieces.
- Turkey and larger birds are often portioned into legs, wings and breasts and then carved into slices separately. Alternatively, the birds can be left whole with the joints separated from the main carcass so as to allow for carving without jointing first.
- Duck usually dissected into four portions: two legs, two wings and the breast cut into long strips down the breast.
- Poussin and small feathered game either serve whole or split into two portions.
- Beef and ham—slice very thinly.
- Joints of lamb, mutton, pork, tongue and veal are usually sliced at double the thickness of beef and ham.
- Boiled beef and pressed meats are generally carved slightly thicker than roast meats, with boiled beef carved with the grain to avoid the meat shredding.
- Lamb best ends are sliced between the cutlet bones and can also be double cut by cutting close to each side of the bone.
- Lamb loin on the bone can be either carved on the bone or removed from the bone and then sliced.
- Rib of beef can either be carved on the bone or by being first removed form the bone and then sliced.

■ Steaks, such as Chateaubriand or double entrecôte, are sliced at angles, either in half, or into more slices depending on guests' preferences.

POTATOES

Examples of potato dishes are:

Airlie: Baked in the oven, emptied out and the mixture blended with butter, cream and spring onions. Refill the skins and sprinkle with grated cheese. Gratinée.

Allemande: Thick sautéd potatoes, which are well buttered.

Alsacienne: New potatoes cooked in butter with bacon and small onions, finish with finely chopped parsley.

Alumettes: Cut into very thin even matchsticks and deep-fried. Dusted with salt when cooked.

Anglaise (à l'): Turned to an even shape and boiled or steamed and seasoned.

Anna: Sliced up, dried and laid into an anna mould with clarified butter and baked.

Au four: Baked potato, washed, pricked and baked on salt, can also be baked in foil. Served in the skin with cross cut in top and flesh pushed upwards. Usually served with butter and pepper mill.

Bataille: Diced and deep-fried.

Berny: Potato croquettes shaped like small apricots combined with tiny chopped truffles. Flour, egg wash and breadcrumbed and mixed with broken sliced almonds. Deep fried.

Berrichonne: Turned, cooked in consommé with finely chopped onions, fine bacon lardons, finished with finely chopped parsley.

Biarritz: Cooked. Mash to a purée with dice of green sweet peppers and herbs added.

Boulangère: Slices of onions and potatoes, cooked in butter, seasoned, moisten with consommé and baked in the oven.

Byron: Macaire covered with grated Chester cheese and cream and gratinated.

Champignol: Fondant potatoes covered with cheese and gratinated.

Château: Turned potatoes, blanched and roasted.

Chips: Wafer thin slices of potato deep fried, dusted with salt when cooked. Also used as roast poultry garnish, known as game chips.

Cocotte: Turned as per château but smaller then roasted.

Crème (à la): (a) Puréed, moistened with milk, butter and seasoning added and serving after adding fresh cream. (b) Peeled and sliced moistened with milk, butter and seasoning added. When serving fresh cream added.

Cretan: Fondante potatoes with powdered thyme.

Croquettes: Prepared as for puréed, combined with egg yolks, formed into an elongated cylinder, panéed and deep fried.

Dauphine: Two parts duchesse potatoes, one part savoury choux paste. Shaped into corks and deep fried.

Dauphinoise: Thinly sliced raw potatoes layered in mould with milk and grated gruyère cheese and then baked in the oven.

Delmonico: Raw dice cooked and then sautéed and browned with breadcrumbs.

Duchesse: Cooked as per purée, thickened with yolks of egg. Piped into walnut whip shape and browned in the oven.

Elizabeth: *Dauphine* with dry purée of spinach.

Fondantes: Large *Château* potatoes, cooked in a white bouillon or consommé so that the top third of the potato is roasted (brush with clarified butter) and the rest is baked with the and the liquid being soaked up into the potato.

Frites: Chipped potatoes, deep fried.

Galette: Duchesse potato in a flat disk or scone shape, criss-cross the top with a knife and coloured in a shallow pan or in the oven.

Gaufrettes: Cut with a mandolin to produce a lattice work effect when sliced, deep fried to golden brown and used as a garnish for game birds.

Gratinées: (a) Well-buttered mashed potatoes, placed in a gratin dish, topped with grated cheese. Gratinée. (b) Baked potatoes halved lengthways the pulp removed and crushed, butter and seasoning is added and the potato mix is placed back into the shells. Top with grated cheese. Gratinée.

Lorette: Dauphine but in a cigar shape.

Lyonnaise: Sautéed potatoes with onions.

Macaire: Shallow-fried floured potato cake made from mashed baked potato pulp, buttered and seasoned.

Maire: As for *à la crème.*

Maître d'hôtel: As for *à la crème* with chopped parsley.

Marquise: Pommes galette with reduced tomato sauce in the mixture.

Menthe: Boiled potatoes with fresh mint in the boiling water.

Mignonette: Allumette but twice the size deep fried.

Mousselline: Mashed potatoes with whipped cream.

Nature: As for *à l'Anglaise* and boiled.

Noisette: Cut with a *noisette* cutter, cooked as per *pommes château.*

Paille: Long julienne cut on a mandolin, dried and deep fried to golden brown, used as part of the garnish for grilled meats.

Parisienne: As for *noisette* but twice the size, roll in meat glaze when finished.

Parmentier: Large roasted cubes of potatoes.

Paysanne: Sliced thickly. Cook in bouillon and butter. Add finely chopped garlic, chiffonade of sorrel and pluches of chervil.

Persillées: à l'Anglaise seasoned and brushed with melted butter and chopped parsley.

Pont-Neuf: Literally *'new bridge'.* From the oldest bridge in Paris where they were originally sold. Pont-Neuf are very large French fried potatoes.

Provençale: Pommes sautées with finely chopped garlic.

Purée: Puréed, seasoned and butter and fresh cream added.

Risolées: As per *château*, but more well browned.

Robe de Chambre: Cooked in water or steamed but in their skins.

Robert: As for *macaire* but with chopped spring onions and eggs.

Rösti: Par-boiled shredded potato with onion seasoning and fried in pan to make large cake.

Sautées: Sliced, par-cooked potatoes, tossed in clarified butter until golden brown and crisp.

Sautées au cru: The same as sautéed, but fried from raw.

Savoyarde: As for *boulangère* but with bacon pieces, and grated cheese on top and then gratinated.

Vapeur: As per *à l'Anglaise*, and steamed.

Villa des Fleurs: As per delmonico with grated gruyère. Gratinée.

Voisin: As for *Anna* with grated cheese.

VEGETABLES

There are an abundant variety of vegetables and preparations. Some of the preparations double up for use with more than one vegetable. Examples of dishes are:

Artichokes (Artichauts)

Argenteuil: Artichoke hearts filled with asparagus tips.

Barigoule: Emptied, stuffed with duxelles, ham and chopped herbs.

Clamart: Hearts with peas and new carrots.

Favorite: Hearts with asparagus tips, mornay sauce, *gratinée* and served with slices of truffles.

Florentine: Hearts garnished with spinach leaves, mornay sauce, *gratinée*.

Gratin: Hearts filled with mornay sauce *gratinée*.

Hollandaise: Cooked complete. Hollandaise served separately.

Italienne: In quarters in butter, covered with italienne sauce.

Paysanne: Quarters in a casserole with pieces of bacon and small onions.

Vinaigrette: *(Cold)* cooked complete and served with separate vinaigrette sauce.

Asparagus (Asperges)

Cold: With a vinaigrette sauce or mayonnaise.

Italienne: As for *milanaise*, without the eggs.

Milanaise: Grated cheese, noisette butter and a fried egg on top.

Mornay: Covered with a mornay sauce, gratinée.

Polonaise: Tips, covered with a noisette butter to which is added chopped shallots, grated hard boiled eggs, breadcrumbs and chopped parsley.

Aubergines (Aubergines / melongène)

Andalouse: In slices, with crushed tomatoes, pimentos and diced ham.

Crème: Cut in rings, sauté, mixed with a cream sauce.

Farcies: Divided into two, fried and stuffed with minced meat, crushed tomatoes, mushrooms and aubergine flesh.

Frites: In thin slices, dipped in flour and fried.

Niçoise: In slices, sautéed in oil with tomatoes, peppers and garlic.

Nimoise: Cut into two and fried, garnished with a tomato, pepper, herb and garlic ragoût.

Provençale: Cut in two, stuffed with breadcrumbs, herbs, garlic and onions.

Baby Marrow (Courgettes)

Crème: Stewed in butter with a light cream sauce.

Farcies: Divided into two, fried and stuffed with duxelles, oven gratinée.

Frites: In thin slices, dipped in flour and fried.

Provençale: Cut in two, stuffed with breadcrumbs herbs, garlic and onions.

Brussels Sprouts (Choux de Bruxelles)

Gratin: Boiled, covered with mornay sauce and gratinée.

Marrons: With butter, garnished with boiled, seasoned and glazed chestnuts.

Velouté: With butter, bound together with velouté sauce.

Cabbage (Choux)

Anglaise: Shredded green cabbage cooked in salt water, strain and well drained, tossed in a little butter and seasoning.

Choucroute: (sauerkraut): Finely shredded. Placed in a braising pan lined with bacon, whole carrots, onion halves, cloves, bunches of mixed herbs, juniper berries and peppercorns in muslin. Moistened with white consommé and white wine. Cooked slowly for 4–5 hours.

Braisés: Washed, blanched, drained and braised with carrots, onions, herbs, and white consommé.

Flamande: Red cabbage, cut into fine julienne, seasoned and cook in a terrine with butter and vinegar and with sugar and a dice of apples added to finish.

Limousine: as above. Moistened with consommé and pieces of raw chestnuts and pork dripping added to finish.

Valencienne: As for *flamande* with chipolatas.

Westphalienne: As for *flamande* with chopped onion tossed in butter moistened with red wine and vinegar.

Cardons, Celery and Fennel (Cardoons, Celeri et Fenouil)

Crème: Stewed in butter with a light cream sauce.

Demi-glace: Stewed with demi-glace sauce.

Gratin: Stewed and covered with mornay sauce, gratinée.

Italienne: Stewed and covered with italienne sauce.

Milanaise: With grated cheese and noisette butter.

Polonaise: Covered with a noisette butter to which is added chopped shallots, grated hard boiled eggs, breadcrumbs and chopped parsley.

Carrots and Turnips (Carottes et Navets)

Chantilly: With cream, peas and butter in the centre.

Crème: Bound with a cream sauce or fresh cream.

Purée: Cooked, puréed, buttered and seasoned and creamed.

Vichy: Sliced, boiled in water and glazed with butter and a little sugar.

Cauliflower and Broccolis (Chou-fleurs et Brocoli)

Anglaise: Boiled, drained and seasoned.

Gratin: Boiled, drained, covered with grated cheese and mornay sauce and gratinated.

Italienne: Boiled, drained, buttered. Coated with tomato flavoured italienne sauce.

Polonaise: Boiled, drained, covered with a noisette butter to which is added chopped shallots, grated hard boiled eggs, breadcrumbs and chopped parsley.

Purée (en): Boiled, drained, passed through a strainer, seasoned and cohered with butter and cream.

Chicory (Endives)

Allemande: Stewed in sour cream and lightly glazed in the oven.

Crème: Stewed and served with cream.

Jus: Stewed in butter and served with the juice.

Mornay: Stewed, covered with mornay sauce, gratinée.

French Beans (Haricots verts)

Allemande: Lightly blanched, drained and sautéed with finely chopped onion cooked in butter with a little flour. Add a little white consommé and finish the cooking in the sauce produced from this process.

Anglaise: Cooked, drained, seasoned and tossed in a little butter.

Crème: Cooked, drained and sautéed in butter and bound with fresh cream.

Maître d'hôtel: Cooked and bound with a light béchamel sauce.

Panachés: Haricots verts and flageolets in equal quantities seasoned and tossed in butter.

Paysanne: Cooked with diced lean bacon and finely chopped onions.

Portugaise: With crushed tomatoes.

Tourangelle: Blanched lightly. Finished in a thin Béchamel sauce with finely chopped garlic and finely chopped parsley.

Japanese Artichokes (Crosnes du Japon)

Crème: Stewed in butter with a light cream sauce, serve in a timbale.

Gratin: Boiled, drained, covered with grated cheese and mornay sauce and gratinated.

Milanaise: Par-boiled, placed on a buttered dish, sprinkled with cheese, melted butter added and glazed and then coated with beurre noisette.

Polonaise: Boiled, drained, covered with a noisette butter to which is added chopped shallots, grated hard boiled eggs, breadcrumbs and chopped parsley.

Purée (en): Boiled, drained, passed through a strainer, seasoned and cohered with butter and cream.

Sautés: Cooked, drained and tossed in very hot butter with seasoning.

Velouté (au): Cooked, drained and cohered with velouté sauce.

Mushrooms (Champignons)

Bordelaise: Cèpes cut in scallops sautéed in oil with finely chopped shallots, finished with finely chopped parsley and lemon juice.

Crème: Stewed in butter and bound with fresh cream.

Croûte: As for *à la crème* but served on croûtons or toasted bread disks.

Gratin: Bound with cream and glazed under the salamander.

Grillés: Button mushrooms basted in oil, season and grilled.

Grillés Bourgignone: As above with snail butter preparation.

Périgourdine: As for *bordelaise* with chopped truffles.

Provençale: Sautéed in oil add herbs, onion and garlic.

Toulousaine: Sliced and tossed in butter, add oil, chopped tomatoes, onions, shallots, garlic and dice of ham.

Tourangelle: Cooked whole in butter, add chopped onions, shallots, garlic and finish with chopped parsley and a little meat glaze to thicken.

Peas and snow peas (Petits pois et Mange-tout (eat-all))

Anglaise (à l'): Boiled in salted water.

Beurre: Boiled, drained and finished with seasonings and butter.

Bonne Femme: À la Française with pieces of bacon and small onions.

Etuvée: A la Française served in an earthenware cocotte dish.

Flamande: With half quantity of new carrots.

Française (à la): Cooked with small onions and chiffonade of lettuce with beurre manié in the stock.

Garniture (purée pour): Three parts purée of peas and one part chicken forcemeat.

Menthe (à la): À l'Anglaise with mint leaves.

Paysanne: A la Française with added paysanne of vegetables.

Purée: Cooked English style, passed through a sieve. Finished with butter and cream.

Spinach (Epinards)

Anglaise (à l'): Boiled leaves, drained and seasoned.

Crème: Boiled leaves drained and squeezed dry. Purée season and bind with fresh cream.

Fleurons: As for *à la crème* but with fleurons around the edge of the spinach.

Oeufs: As for *à la crème* but with quarters of hard boiled eggs around the outside.

Tomatoes (Tomates)

Ancienne: Stuffed with duxelles with added ham and herbs.

Concassées: Blanched and cut up into small cubes stewed in butter, tomato paste, white wine, seasoning, with finely chopped shallots and onions.

Farcies: As per *ancienne* but covered with breadcrumbs and grilled.

Grillé: Brushed with melted butter seasoned and grilled under the salamander.

Italienne: Stuffed with italienne risotto.

Provençale: Cut up, cooked in the oven with breadcrumbs, garlic, chopped parsley and seasoning.

SALADS AND SALAD DRESSINGS

Salads have fairly distinct groupings according to the range of ingredients used and their method of preparation:

Crudités

Crudités are generally eaten with the fingers, as an hors-d'oeuvre at the start of a meal. They are accompanied with a variety of dressings, sauces purées and salsas into which they are dipped. Examples of crudités are:

- Small cauliflower florets
- Hearts of celery with leaf attached
- Pimentos of various colours in julienne
- Whole peeled baby carrots with their fresh tops
- Spring onions
- Cherry tomatoes
- Radishes turned into flowers

- Baby fennel
- Cucumber

Simple salads

These tend to be composed of but one, or at most, a very few raw ingredients. These can be dressed and garnished, examples are:

Simple green salad	Crisp, fresh green lettuce leaves or hearts. Tossed in vinaigrette at the table (purpose: to refresh the palate after the main course).
Green salad	Selected or a selection of green leaves, cucumber, spring onions, cucumber, green pimentos, baby spinach, chervil etc.
Mixed salad	As above with other flavouring elements such as chicory, tomatoes, dandelion.
Tomato salad	Plum tomato salad, or other variety, served with a light or contrasting dressing.
Cucumber salad	Light, crisp and fresh.
Celery ravé	Shredded celery possibly with a light nut and apple dressing.
Watercress	To add a peppery note.

Mixed salads

The crudités and simple salads lend themselves to being mixed together.

Cooked vegetables for salads

Some vegetables are inedible or difficult to digest raw whilst others are quite simply enhanced by cooking. Some vegetables, including green and dried French and runner beans, broad beans and selected pulses must be cooked, as they are toxic in varying degrees when raw. Examples of cooked vegetables used in salads are:

- Beetroot
- Jerusalem artichoke
- Parsnip
- Potatoes
- Salsify
- Scorzonera

Marinated salads

Marinades are often liquids which are either highly or subtly flavoured, often spiced or herbed. Vinaigrette is the most common marinade for vegetables, but lemon juice, vinegar, or oil whether flavoured or not are also used. Some vegetables have the sort of texture that easily absorbs marinades. The vegetables acquire a particular balance/texture/flavour/aroma profile as a result. Examples are:

- Peppers
- Grated carrots
- Globe artichoke
- Leeks
- Aubergines
- Cabbage

Compound salads

These are complex mixed salads. Examples include:

Aïda: Curly chicory, tomatoes, slices of artichoke bottoms, julienne of green pimentos and whites of hard boiled eggs, cover with hard yolks passed through a sieve, vinaigrette and mustard.

Américaine: Sliced tomatoes and potatoes, julienne of celery, onions and hard boiled eggs, vinaigrette.

Andalouse: Quarters of tomatoes, julienne of sweet pimentos , boiled rice, crushed garlic, onions and chopped parsley, vinaigrette.

Béatrice: Julienne of white of chicken , truffles, potatoes, asparagus tips, sauce mayonnaise with mustard.

Caesar: Salad of cos (or Romaine) lettuce, dressed with vinaigrette (originally containing near raw egg yolk) or other similar dressing, garlic, croûtons and grated (or shaved) Parmesan cheese. Additional ingredients include anchovies paste to flavour the dressing or put in whole fillets into the salad.

Caprise de Reine: Chicory, apples, julienne of celery and truffles, mayonnaise sauce.

Châtelaine: Hard boiled eggs, truffles, artichoke bottoms, potatoes, vinaigrette with chopped tarragon.

Créole: Small melons scoop out the inside cut in small dice, add salt and ginger, rice mixed with acidulated cream, replace in the melon. Serve surrounded by crushed ice.

Cressonière: Slices of potatoes, watercress leaves, sprinkle with parsley, chervil and hard boiled eggs.

Delmonico: Celeriac and apples in dice, bound lightly in mayonnaise thinned with cream.

Demi-deuil: Julienne of truffles and potatoes, border round with slices of each, cream and mustard.

Florida: Lettuces and quarters of oranges seasoned with acidulated cream.

Grand-duchese: French beans, julienne of potatoes and celery. Mayonnaise.

Indienne: Rice, asparagus tips, julienne of sweet pimentos, dice of apples, curry cream.

Italiene: Vegetable salad with small dice of salami and fillets of anchovies, mayonnaise.

Jockey-Club: Asparagus tips, truffles, mayonnaise.

Lorette: Mace, celery, beetroot, vinaigrette.

Mascotte: Asparagus tips, hard boiled eggs, peeled shrimps, truffles, mustard and cream.

Mignonettes: Large brunoise chopped vegetables, salad mayonnaise.

Mimosa: Lettuce hearts, oranges, grapes, bananas, cream and lemon juice.

Monégasque: Potatoes, quarter artichokes, tomatoes, black olives. Mustard sauce and anchovies.

Niçoise: French beans, tomatoes, potatoes, anchovy fillets, olives, capers, vinaigrette.

Opéra: Chicken breasts, celery, truffles, tongue, asparagus tips, gherkins. Light mayonnaise.

Parisienne: Slices of crayfish, truffles, Russian salad, bound with mayonnaise and aspic.

Rachel: Celery, truffles, artichoke hearts, asparagus tips, potatoes. Light mayonnaise.

Russe: Carrots, turnips, peas, potatoes, in macedoine cut, French beans, Mayonnaise.

Saint Sylvestre: Celeriac, artichoke mushroom and truffle salad.

Tosca: Chicken, celery, truffles, mayonnaise.

Tourangelle: Potatoes, french beans, broad beans. Mayonnaise made with cream and chopped tarragon.

Waldorf: Apples, celery, walnuts, mayonnaise.

Salad dressings

Salad dressings come in many widely differing permutations. In addition to **vinaigrette and derivatives** (see page 118) and **mayonnaise and derivatives** (see page 117), other examples include:

- *Anchovy:* Finely chopped anchovies, dry English mustard, vegetable oil, olive oil, white wine vinegar and pepper.

- *Spicy:* Vegetable oil, white wine vinegar, paprika, Dijon mustard, chilli sauce.

- *Egg:* Hard boiled egg finely mashed, capers finely chopped, finely chopped pickled cucumber, vegetable oil, white vinegar, finely chopped parsley, finely chopped chives.

- *Fresh herb:* English dry mustard, vegetable oil, white vinegar, finely chopped parsley, finely chopped chervil, finely chopped chives, finely chopped French tarragon.

- *Blue cheese:* Blue cheese, cream, vegetable oil, white wine vinegar, pepper, lemon juice.

The various oils, vinegars and mustards include:

Oils

- Olive
- Safflower
- Sunflower
- Grape seed
- Groundnut
- Hazelnut
- Peanut oil
- Soya
- Sesame
- Walnut oil

Vinegars

- Wine vinegar
- Cider vinegar
- Sherry vinegar
- Flavoured vinegars

Mustards

- English
- French
- Dijon
- Meaux
- Herb
- German

CHEESE

One of the most ancient forms of processed food. Cheese is available in manufactured and artisanal forms. Artisinal cheese is usually made with milk from the cheese-maker's own herd. In this way cheese makers can assure the highest quality of their own materials. There is less uniformity and more autonomy over the cheese making process, almost impossible in factory conditions.

Service of cheese

For best results the cheese should be allowed to temperature by being left out of the fridge for at least one hour before serving. Cheese can be stored in a cool place such as a cellar or fridge but should be wrapped in aluminium foil to prevent it from drying out.

Cheese is usually served either by itself or with various breads or biscuits being offered. Butter or an alternative is also sometimes expected. Radishes and celery may also be offered, as may fresh fruit such as grapes, apples or pears. Sometimes salad is also provided. Salt is provided for the celery and caster sugar for cream cheeses. The cover is either a side knife and sweet fork, if the cheese is to be eaten from the plate, or a side knife and side plate if the cheese is being eaten with biscuits or bread.

Accompaniments for cheese include:

- salt, pepper, mustard
- assorted cheese biscuits, crackers, sweet digestive biscuits, water biscuits, Ryvita, crispbreads

- butter and/or alternatives
- assorted breads—the more delicate the cheese, the whiter and less salted the bread accompaniment. Powerful blue cheeses can handle spiced breads made with sour milk already containing a dairy flavour
- speciality breads such as Pain Poilâne
- stringed slivers of celery served in a glass part filled with crushed ice on an under-plate
- caster sugar (with cream cheeses)
- radishes, when in season, placed in a glass bowl on under-plate with teaspoon

Types and examples of cheese

Cheeses are distinguished by flavour and categorized according to their texture. They differ from each other for a number of reasons, mainly arising through variations in the making process. Differences occur in the rind and how it is formed, in the paste, and in the cooking (both time and temperature). Additionally cheeses vary because the milk used comes from different animals: cow, sheep, or goat.

The texture of a cheese depends largely on the period of maturation, the main categories being:

- fresh (eaten within a few days of being made)
- soft
- semi-hard
- hard
- blue cheeses

Fresh Cheese

Bigoton: French, Loire, goat's milk cheese. It is small, oval and sold approximately one week old. It is dusted with ash and has a fresh lemony taste and very light texture which melts in the mouth. As it matures it becomes wrinkled and develops a grey rind. At this point it becomes goaty and runny.

Brocciu, Broccio AOC: Produced in the départements of Cors-du-Sud and Haute Corse. This is a whey cheese from goat's and cow's milk.

Cottage: Unripened low-fat, skimmed milk cheese with a granular curd. Originated in the United States of America and now has many variations.

Cream: Similar to cottage cheese but is made with full-fat milk. There are a number of different varieties available, some made from non-cows milk.

Feta: Traditionally made with ewe's milk.

Fromage frais: Cow's goat's and sheep's milk French cheese. An ancient cheese dating back thousands of years. Both artisanal and factory produced versions are made. Literally—'fresh cheese'. Describes a group of cheeses which are unripened, mousse like consistency/texture, have high moisture content with a citrus zing on the palate. Fat content can vary widely from: maigre—very low 5 per cent—to allége—double and triple crème 75 per cent. The names can vary widely Fontainbleau, Chèvre Frais, Faiselle de Chèvre, Fromage Blanc, Petit Swiss etc.

Mozzarella: Italian cheese made now from cow's milk but originally from buffalo milk.

Quark: Continental version of cottage cheese, sharper and more acidic than the American versions. Mainly German and Austrian varieties available..

Ricotta: Italian cheese made from the whey of cow's milk. A number of other Italian varieties are available made from sheep's milk

Soft Cheese

Barbery, Fromage de Troyes: French cheese similar to Camembert but sometimes sold unripened as a fresh cheese.

Bel Paese: A light and creamy Italian cheese has a name which means 'beautiful country'.

Brie: Famous French cheese made since the eighth century. Other countries now make this style of cheese, distinguishing it by their country's name e.g., Scottish Brie.

Brie de Meaux AOC: French cow's milk from the Ile-de-France. This cheese stands out amongst other Brie cheeses. It is smooth, creamy but not quite runny and scented with mushrooms. The earliest record of this cheese is from AD774. Well worth the investment.

Brillat-Savarin: A triple cream cow's milk cheese. When young it melts in the mouth and has a buttery slightly sour taste. As its velvety crust appears it becomes more tangy.

Camembert: Famous French cheese which is stronger and can be more pungent than Brie.

Camembert de Normandie AOC: Famous French cow's milk cheese. Only cheese-makers in Calvados, Eure, Manche, Orne and Seine Maritime are permitted to use the term 'Camembert de Normandie AOC'. It has a scent to it of wild mushrooms. It has a delicious creamy consistency.

Coulommiers: A small version of Brie. Similar to Brie de Meaux. It has a lovely texture and mushroom aroma, but milder.

Epoisses: French Burgundian cheese, speciality of the area. Sometimes dipped in Marc de Bourgogne (local brandy) before being sold.

Explorateur: French cow's milk cheese enriched with cream. A small cylinder with a white downy surface, invented in the 1950s. So named in honour of 'Explorer' the first satellite to be launched by the USA.

Feta: Greek cheese made from both goat's and sheep's milk.

Gaperon: French cow's milk cheese from the Auvergne with garlic and spicy peppercorns.

Gratte Paille: Almost twice the thickness of Camembert. This cow's milk cheese from the Ile-de-France is enriched with cream. Long ripening means that most still have a slight chalkiness in the centre, but are smooth and rich towards the outside. As the interior ages and develops a pleasant sharpness can be evidenced.

Straccihino: Italian cheese originally from Lombardy. A softy, delicate cheese which now has a number of varieties.

Semi-Hard Cheese

Appenzeller: Typical example of Swiss cheese textures. The name is from the Latin for 'abbot's cell'.

Caerphilly: Buttermilk-flavoured cheese with a soft taste. Originally a Welsh cheese but now manufactured all over Britain.

Cantal: French cheese from the Auvergne, similar to Cheddar.

Cheddar: Classic British cheese now made all over the world and referred to as, for example, Scottish Cheddar, Canadian cheddar etc.

Cheshire: Crumbly, slightly salty cheese, available as either white or red. It was originally made during the 12th century in Cheshire but is now made all over Britain.

Chèvre: The name means 'goat', which denotes the origin of the milk from which this cheese, and the wide variety of variations, is made.

Derby: English Derbyshire cheese now more often known by the sage-flavoured variety, Sage Derby.

Dunlop: This Scottish cheese is similar to cheddar and is said to have come from an Irish recipe.

Edam: Similar to, but harder than, Gouda this Dutch cheese has a buttery taste and a yellow or red wax coated rind. It is sometimes flavoured with cumin.

Emmenthal: The name of this Swiss cheese refers to the Emme Valley. It is similar to Gruyère although it is softer.

Esrom: Similar to the French, Port Salut, this Danish cheese has a red rather than yellow rind.

Gloucester/Double: Full-cream, classic English cheeses originally Gloucester made only from the milk of Gloucestershire cows.

Gouda: Buttery textured, soft and mild flavoured well-known Dutch cheese with a yellow or red rind.

Gruyère: Mainly known as a Swiss cheese, but both French and Swiss varieties can be legally called by this name. It has small pea-size holes and a smooth relatively hard texture. The French varieties have larger holes.

Jarlsberg: Similar to Emmenthal, this Norwegian cheese was first produced in the late 1950s. It has a yellow wax coating.

Lancashire: Another classic English cheese similar to Cheshire; (white Cheshire is sometimes sold as Lancashire).

Leicester: Mild flavoured and orange coloured cheese.

Limberger: Often quite pungent, this, originally Belgian, cheese is now also available from Germany.

Manchego: Relatively hard cheese which may have holes and has either a white or sometimes yellow paste. Made in Spain from sheep's milk.

Monterey: Creamy, soft American cheese with many holes. A harder version known as Monterey Jack is suitable for grating.

Mysost: Similar Gjetost, this Norwegian cheese has a firm consistency and a sweetish taste.

Pont l'Evêque: Similar to Camembert, but square in shape, this French cheese originates from Normandy.

Port Salut: Mild flavoured cheese with a name meaning 'Port of Salvation', referring to the abbey where exiled Trappist monks returned after the French Revolution.

Reblochon: Creamy, mild flavoured cheese from the Haute-Savoie region of France. The name comes from the illegal 'second milking' from which the cheese was originally made.

Samso: Originally made on the Dutch island of the same name as a copy of the Swiss Emmenthal cheese. There are now many variations.

Tilsit: Strong flavoured cheese from the East German town of the same name where it was first produced by Dutch living there. Now available from other parts of Germany.

Wensleydale: Yorkshire cheese originally made from sheep's or goat's milk but now from cow's milk. This cheese is the traditional accompaniment to apple pie.

Hard Cheese

Bergkäse: Smooth, mild flavoured cheese from Austria.

Caciocavallo: Originating from ancient Roman times, the name means 'cheese on horseback' because its shape is said to resemble saddlebags.

Kefalotyri: Literally Greek for 'hard cheese', this is a tasty, grating-type cheese from Greece.

Parmesan: Classic Italian hard cheese, more correctly called Parmigiano Reggiano, and predominantly known as the grated cheese used in, and for sprinkling over, Italian dishes.

Pecorino: Hard sheep's milk, grating or table cheese from southern Italy. Also available with added peppercorns as Pecorino Pepato from Sicily.

Provolone: Smoked cheese made in America, Australia, and Italy. Now made from cow's milk but originally from buffalo milk. Younger versions are softer and milder than the longer kept varieties.

Blue Cheese

Bavarian Blue: Rich, delicious high fat and slightly sourish German cheese.

Bleu d'Auvergne: French, Auvergne cheese which becomes blue through the addition of Penicillium glaucum mould. As the interior of the maturing cheese starts to collapse, the flavour intensifies to a ripe spicy tang.

Bleu de Bresse: Fairly soft and mild flavoured French cheese from the area between Soane-et-Loire and the Jura.

Blue Cheshire: One of the finest blue cheeses which only becomes blue accidentally, although the makers endeavour to assist this process by prickling the cheese and maturing it in a favourable atmosphere.

Bresse Bleu: French, Rhône-Alpes, cow's milk cheese. Brie style and with the blue injected into the cheese, which leaves pockets of blue grey mould rather than the more common spidery mould.

Cashel Blue: Irish cheese from County Tipperary, Cow's milk. In youth it is firm and crumbly but gradually it mellows and becomes creamier. Quite strong but well worth the investment, made by Jane and Louis Grubb.

Cambazola: German cow's milk Brie style cheese created in the 1970s. This is a quality cheese an amalgamation of Camembert and Gorgonzola as the name and style hints. Spicy sweet/sour subtle taste. Excellent for those who are connoisseurs, but might not otherwise try a blue cheese.

Danish Blue: One of the most well-known of the blue cheeses. Softish and mild flavoured, it was one of the first European blue cheeses to gain popularity in Britain.

Dolcelatte: Factory made version of Gorgonzola. The name is Italian for 'sweet milk' and the cheese is fairly soft with a creamy texture and greenish veining.

Fourme d'Ambert: The oldest blue cheese in France. It is not high in salt like some other blue cheeses. It is creamy, soft and unctuous. The blue is natural and not injected.

Gorgonzola: Softish sharp flavoured, classic Italian cheese with green veining, which is developed with the addition of mould culture.

Lanark Blue: Humphrey Errington makes this lovely Lanarkshire, Scottish sheep's milk unpasteurized cheese. Aromatic herbaceous and rich moist blue, a connoisseurs cheese.

Roquefort: Classic, sheep's milk cheese from the southern Massif Central in France. The maturing takes place in caves which provide a unique humid environment which contributes to the development of the veining.

Stilton: Famous and classic English cheese made from cow's milk. The white Stilton has also become popular and is slightly less flavoursome than the blue variety.

SWEETS

The range of possible sweets is very extensive and varied. There are no particular accompaniments to sweets. Most sweets are generally served onto sweet plates or are pre-plated with puddings and various hot dishes being be pre-plated, or served into, various bowls. The choice of whether to serve on a plate or in a bowl is dependent on the texture of the sweet dish, e.g. fruit salad in a bowl and gâteau on a plate.

The lay-up is usually the sweet spoon and fork. Often the customer may require a sugar sifter. Various items may require different cutlery for instance a sundae spoon, ice cream spoon or teaspoon. The main consideration is always to aid eating.

Cut gateaux or flans are served on plates and placed so that the pointed end is towards the customer. The serving of sauces, e.g. custard, and whipped cream can be out of sauceboats (spooned not poured) or there may be individual portion jugs. Alternatively the sauceboats may be left (on an underplate) on the table for the customers to help themselves. If sauces are served then it is usual not to serve these over the item but around it—unless the customer specifically requests it.

Examples of sweet dishes:

Bavarois and mousses (cold)

Mousse based on milk, egg yolks, sugar, vanilla, gelatine and whipped cream with various flavourings: chocolate, lemon, coffee, orange, kirsch, etc. Moulded to various shapes.

Bombes

Ice cream preparations made into bomb shapes using moulds. Examples are:

Africaine: Vanilla bombe covered in chocolate ice.

Aida: Kirsch bombe, coated with strawberry ice.

Alhambra: Strawberry bombe, coated with vanilla ice.

Brésilienne: Pineapple ice outside, vanilla and rum bombe inside.

Marie-Louise: Chocolate ice outside, vanilla bombe inside.

Tortoni: Praline ice outside, coffee bombe inside.

Tutti Frutti: Strawberry ice outside, lemon and preserved fruit bombe inside.

Charlottes (cold)

Chantilly: A mould lined with sponge fingers and filled with chantilly cream.

Mont reuil: A mould lined with sponge fingers, filled with a kirsch flavoured bavarian cream and garnished with peaches.

Napolitaine: A mould lined with genoise biscuits, scooped out and filled with chestnut purée and chantilly cream.

Russe: A mould lined with sponge fingers, half filled with a vanilla flavoured bavarois and half with chantilly cream.

Charlottes hot

Apple: Slices of bread, laid in a mould with diced apple between them. Cooked in the oven and removed from the mould.

Coupes (served in coupe, or sundae, dishes)

Alexandra: Mixed fruit in kirsch with strawberry ice.

Belle Hélène: Vanilla ice, half a pear covered with chocolate sauce.

Bresilienne: Pineapple cubes with maraschino and lemon ice.

Jacques: Mixed fruit with kirsch, lemon and strawberry ice.

Jamaïque: Pineapple and rum, coffee ice.

Melba: Vanilla ice, half a peach covered with a raspberry (Melba) sauce.

Montmorency: Cherries in kirsch, vanilla ice.

Romanoff: Vanilla ice garnished with strawberries flavoured with liqueur and mixed with chantilly cream.

Royale: Mixed fruit in kirsch, vanilla ice.

Tutti Frutti: Fruit preserved in kirsch, strawberry, pineapple and lemon ice

Creams (Crèmes)

Anglaise: (Custard), consisting of milk, sugar, vanilla and eggs (served hot or cold).

Beau-Rivage: An edging of caramel cream around cornets filled with chantilly cream.

Brûlée: Thick smooth and rich baked custard with a covering of caramelised sugar.

Caprice: Chantilly cream to which crushed meringues have been added.

Caramel: A mixture consisting of milk, sugar, eggs and vanilla, cooked in a charlotte mould in which a caramel has been formed.

Diverses: Custards with various flavourings, such as chocolate, coffee, praline, lemon, etc.

Printanière: Chantilly cream with strawberry puree.

Renversée: The same as caramel cream.

Fritters (beignets) (hot)

Fruits: Such as pineapple, apple, banana, etc., dipped in batter and deep-fried.

Marie-Louise: Rounds of choux pastry added to preserved fruits and fried.

Souffles: Small balls of puff pastry, fried.

Fruit salads

Various citrus, soft fruit, tropical and stoned fruits in various cuts served chilled either on their own, with stock syrups, with liqueur, rosewater, mint and various other flavouring ingredients.

Fruit sweets (cold)

Alma: Pears poached in Port wine, garnish with grilled almond powder and decorated with whipped cream.

Almina: Tangerines bavarois with kirsch placed back into the tangerine shell with the lid place back on top. Decorated with crystallised violets.

Cardinal: Strawberries, peaches and pears, poached and laid on vanilla ice cream and coated with raspberry purée. Garnished with grilled sliced almonds.

Château-Lafitte: Peaches in halves poached in wine and sugar. Syrup is reduced with raspberry and red currant jelly and poured over.

Compote: Various fruits peeled and poached in a light stock syrup flavoured to taste.

Créole: Strawberries macerated in kirsch and maraschino. Served on thin slices of pineapple.

Fool: All sorts of fruits poached in syrup, passed through a sieve and then blended with whipped cream.

Jelly: Either proprietary, or made fresh and set with gelatine, and either plain or with fruits set within.

Marquise: Strawberries lightly macerated in kirsch, then drained and rolled in castor sugar, laid on whipped cream mixed with strawberry purée.

Melba: Strawberries, nectarines, peaches, pears laid on vanilla ice and coated with raspberry purée. Draped with spun sugar.

Ritz: Strawberries coated with chantilly cream mixed with half purée of strawberries and half purée of raspberries.

Romanoff: Strawberries soaked in curaçao, coated with whipped cream.

Wilhelmine: Strawberries macerated in kirsch orange and sugar. Served with vanilla whipped cream.

Fruit sweets (hot)

Andalouse: Apricots, pineapple, peaches, apples, pears. Poached and laid on vanilla ice cream, coat and decorate with Italian meringue, serve pink fruit syrup apart.

Beurre: Apples with the middles scooped out and refilled, with butter and vanilla syrup cooked in the oven. Coated with buttered apricot sauce.

Bonne Femme: Apples with the middles scooped out and refilled, with butter and sugar.

Cardinal: Pears or apples, cut into quarters and poached in sugar syrup. Sauce is made with reduce stock and crème de cassis. Decorated with fresh chopped walnuts.

Cerises Jubilée: Poached stoned cherries, reduce caramelised cooking liquor is flambéed with brandy or kirsch.

Château-Lafitte: Peaches in halves poached in wine and sugar. Coated with sauce made with reduced syrup with raspberry and red currant jelly.

Compôte: Various fruits peeled and poached in a light stock syrup flavoured to taste (can be served cold).

Condé: Apricots, pineapple, bananas, peaches, pears or apples, poached and dressed on creamed rice and coated with thickened syrup or apricot jam.

Feu d'Enfer: All kinds of fruits, poached and flamed with liqueur to taste.

Gâteaux

Chocolat: Chocolate génoise with chocolate cream or buttercream.

Forêt Noir: Black forest: chocolate génoise with cream, kirsch, stoned black cherries or morello cherries and chocolate shavings.

Moka: Coffee génoise with coffee cream or buttercream.

Printanière: Génoise buttercream ⅓ coloured green and flavoured with almond essence, ⅓ pink and with raspberry essence and ⅓ plain. Each of the three layers of the gâteau are spread with a different buttercream with the top and the sides are covered in plain buttercream and toasted almonds. The top is decorated with small roses of each coloured buttercream.

St Honoré: Choux pastry gateau filled with fruits and whipped garnished with choux pastry buns filled with crème St Honoré, glace fruits and spun sugar topping.

Ices

Ices take various forms, are dressed in various ways and sometimes mixed together. Examples include:

Biscuit glacé: Egg yolk, sugar, whisked egg whites, whipped cream and various flavourings.

Bombe glacé: Egg yolks, sugar syrup, whipped cream and various flavourings.

Glace crème: Egg yolks, milk, sugar, cream and various flavours.

Glace aux fruits: Fruit pulp, sugar syrup and lemon juice.

Parfait glacé: The same arrangement as for a bombe.

Sorbet: Sugar syrup, white wine or champagne, orange or lemon juice and peel. Any sorbet can be named according to the ingredients, such as: vanilla, mocha, coffee, chocolate, lemon, apricot, pineapple, strawberry, mandarin, nut, orange, peach, pistachio, etc., together with the various liqueurs.

Omlettes

Confitures: An omelette mixed with jam and glazed under a red-hot grill.

Norvégienne or surprise: A génoise sponge base garnished with ice and covered with a *soufflé* omelette mixture, decorated and placed in a very hot oven for a short period.

Rhum: Covered with sugar, glazed under a red hot grill, covered with rum and *flambé* at the table.

Soufflée: A mixture of sugar, egg yolks and various flavourings stirred into egg whites that have been whipped until they are firm. Placed on an oval dish, decorated with a confectioner's syringe and slowly cooked in the oven.

Stéphanie: Omelette cooked as a *soufflé* in the pan and stuffed with a hot mixture of fruits flavoured with kirsch.

Pancakes (Crêpes) (hot)

Georgette: Stuffed with kirsch flavoured pineapple.

Gil-Blas: Flavoured with lemon, stuffed with hazelnut butter.

Normande: Stuffed with diced apple.

Suzette: Flavoured with orange, stuffed with pommade butter to which the peel and juice of an orange have been added, curaçao and brandy.

Pastry items (pies, flans and other pastries)

Bakewell Tart: Sugar pastry tart filled with raspberry jam base topped with frangipane filling, when baked this is apricot glazed, and finally coated with water icing.

Bande aux fruits: Either puff pastry-based or sugar pastry-based with either crème pâtissière or crème frangipane with fresh fruits on top and glazed.

Flan: Sugar or short pastry-based with crème piatissière and fruit topping glazed, e.g. aux pêches, aux poires, aux pommes, aux framboises etc.

Lemon meringue pie: Sugar pastry base with deep lemon middle and baked meringue topping.

Mille-feuille: Thin layers of puff pastry, spread with raspberry jam and crème pâtissière. The top is brushed with apricot glaze and then covered in fondant, thin chocolate is run out over the top and this is made into a decorative shape, toasted flaked almonds also feature.

Sacher Torte: Very rich chocolate cake with apricot filling.

Tarte Tatin: Half-peeled and cored apples cooked with sugar and butter in a pan topped with sweet pastry and baked. Turned out onto a serving dish and glazed with apricot jam.

Puddings

Bread and butter: Thin slices of bread spread with butter, with currants, covered in egg custard and baked.

Brésilien: Ground tapioca pudding, cooked in a mould in which a caramel has been made.

Cabinet: Made in a charlotte mould with pieces of Génoise sponge, preserved fruit, a covering of egg custard and baked, served hot.

Egg Custard: Cooked in a pudding dish and flavoured to taste.

Diplomate: The same as a *cabinet* pudding but served cold with redcurrant, raspberry, apricot or vanilla sause.

Maltais: Pudding flavoured with orange and with an orange sauce.

Montmorency: Pudding made from cherries preserved in kirsch and a fruit sauce.

Plum pudding (Christmas pudding): Bread crumbs, suet, raisins, preserved fruit, rum, etc. flambé with rum at the table, served with white rum or brandy sauce or brandy butter.

Royal: A soufflé lemon pudding with biscuits.

Saxon: A soufflé pudding flavoured with lemon and vanilla.

Soufflés

A soufflé is a mixture consisting of flour, sugar, milk, butter and egg yolk, mixed into egg whites that are whipped stiff and then cooked slowly in the oven. The soufflé is generally flavoured with various flavourings such as: lemon, chocolate, orange, pineapple, strawberry, cherry, banana, coffee, various liqueurs, etc.

Syllabubs

These are made of sugar, eggs, white wine, Marsala, port or champagne, all mixed together when hot to obtain a sort of frothy light cream.

SAVOURIES

On the lunch and dinner menu a savoury may generally be served as an alternative to sweet. In a banquet it may be a separate course served in addition to either a sweet or cheese course.

Savouries may be:

- Canapés or croûtes—shaped pieces of bread about 6mm(¼in) thick, brushed with melted butter and grilled, or may be shaped shallow fried bread.

- On toast—usually shaped pieces of toast with various toppings such as anchovies, sardines, mushrooms, smoked haddock, and the classic Welsh, or Buck rarebit.

- In tartlets or in bouchées—where fillings are either heaped or piped into tartlets, barquettes (boat shapes) or bouchée (literally means 'mouthful') and these comprise small light pastry or vol-au-vents filled with an array of savoury mixtures.

- Quiche—savoury egg tartlets such as the famous Quiche Lorraine or Alsace onion quiches and tarts.
- Omelettes—a selection of savoury omelettes can be drawn from the egg section and utilised here.
- Soufflés—savoury soufflés such as the classic cheese or broccolis, Parmesan, haddock, spinach etc. can also be served as savouries.

Savoury items can also be placed into glass dishes as in the *classic champignons sous cloche*—mushrooms filled with *beurre maître d' hôtel*—parsley butter and cooked slowly under the glass cover. The savoury aroma to be released in front of the guest at the table.

Cover, accompaniments and service

The main cover for a savoury is usually a side knife and a sweet fork. Accompaniments are:

- Salt and pepper
- Cayenne pepper
- Pepper mill
- Worcestershire sauce (usually only with meat savouries)

Savouries are usually pre-portioned by the kitchen and served onto a hot fish plate. The savoury is served plated to the guest after the cover and accompaniments have been placed on the table.

Examples of savouries:

Canapés:

Charlemagne: Shrimps in a curry sauce.

Champignons: English mushrooms seasoned and grilled.

Diablotin: Garnish small gnoki, sprinkle with cheese and glaze.

Ecossais: Scrambled eggs with an anchovy fillet in the middle as garnish.

Epicure: Roquefort cheese with butter and chopped dry walnuts piled into a canapé.

Fédora: Grilled mushrooms and bacon with a stuffed olive.

Gourmets (des): Chopped ham seasoned and blended with mustard butter.

Haddock: Fillets of haddock cooked in butter flaked and placed on to a canapé.

Hollandaise: Chopped haddock and slices of hard boiled eggs.

Ritchie: Chopped haddock cooked in cream, sprinkled with cheese and glazed under the salamander.

Quo Vadis: Grilled roes garnished with small mushrooms

Croûtes:

Croque Monsieur: Slices of cooked ham placed between two slices of gruyère cheese, then between two slices of thin plain bread. Cut with a round cutter and shallow fry both sides in clarified butter.

Croûte Derby: Ham purée placed on a croûte garnished with a pickled walnut and parsley en branche.

Croûte Diane: Chicken livers wrapped in streaky bacon on a skewer and grilled.

Ivanhoe: Purée of haddocks cooked in cream with a small grilled mushroom on top.

Radjah: Ham purée with curry topped with chutney.

Windsor: Ham paste. Cover with grilled mushrooms.

Toasts:

Anges à Cheval: Angels on horseback. Bearded Poached oysters wrapped in thin slices of bacon. Skewer and grill. Served on toast.

Buck rarebit: As above topped with a poached egg.

Sardines: Skinned and boned sardines dusted with cayenne pepper.

Scotch woodcock: Scrambled eggs on toast, topped with a trellis of anchovies studded with capers.

Welsh rarebit: Melt cheddar cheese with cream and beer, cayenne pepper and Lea and Perrins sauce, egg yolks and Béchamel. Spread on toast and glaze under the salamander.

Tartlets and Barquettes:

Eureka: *(Barquettes)* mushroom soufflé garnished with an anchovy.

Favorite: *(Tartlets)* parmesan soufflé with dice of truffles and crayfish tails.

Florentine: *(Tartlets)* spinach in leaves, parmesan soufflé and anchovy purée.

Marquise: *(Tartlets)* the sides of the tartlets are coated in gnoki paste the centre filled with Mornay sauce and cayenne pepper.

Raglan: *(Tartlets)* smoked herring roe purée covered with haddock soufflé.

Tosca: *(Tartlets)* crayfish cooked American style covered covered with parmesan soufflé.

FRESH FRUIT (DESSERT)

The term 'dessert' traditionally only referred to fresh fruit and nuts (although nowadays the term is used to refer to sweets generally). On an à la carte menu, fresh fruit and nuts was often a section on its own and it included all types of fresh fruits and nuts according to season. However the majority of the more popular items are available all the year round, due to the up-to-date means of transport between various parts of the world. Sometimes candied fruits are included in the fruit basket.

The lay-up for dessert (fresh fruit and nuts) is:

- Fruit plate
- Fruit knife and fork
- Finger bowl and spare napkin
- Debris plate
- Nutcracker and grape scissors, placed in fruit basket
- Caster sugar dredger on table
- Salt cellar for nuts

Types of fruits

Soft Fruits

Blackberries	*la mûre de ronce*
Blackcurrants	*le cassis*
Gooseberries	*la groseille à macquereau*
Loganberries	*La ronce-framboise*
Raspberries	*la framboise*
Red currants	*les groseilles rouge*
Strawberries	*la fraises*
White currants	*les groseille blanche*
Bilberry	*la myrtille*

Stone Fruits

Apricots	*l'abricot*
Cherries	*la cerises*
Coconut	*La noix de coco*
Damsons	*la prune de damas*
Greengages	*la reine-claude*
Mangoes	*la mangue*
Nectarines	*la nectarine*
Peaches	*la pêche*
Plums	*la prune*
Pear/avocado	*l'avocat*
Papaya	*la papaye*
Lychee	*le lytchee*

Hard Fruits

Apples	*la pomme*
Pears	*la poire*

Citrus Fruits

Clementines	*la clémentine*
Grapefruits	*la pamplemouse*
Lemons	*le citron*
Limes	*Le citron vert; le limette*
Mandarines	*la mandarine*
Oranges	*l'orange*
Pink grapefruits	*la pamplemousse rosé*
Sanguine oranges (blood oranges)	*la sanguine*
Satsumas	*la satsuma*
Tangerines	*la mandarine*

Tropical and Other

Bananas	*la banane*
Cranberries	*les aireles*
Dates	*la datte*
Figs	*la figue*
Grapes	*les raisins*
Jackfruit	*Le ti Jacque*
Kiwi	*le kiwi*
Longan	*le logane*
Melons	*le melon*
Passion fruit	*Le fruit de la passion*
Paw Paws	*la patte de patte*
Pineapple	*l'ananas*
Rhubarb	*la rhubarbe*
Tomatillo	*la physallis*
Plantain	*la banane plantain*
Pomegranate	*la grenade*

Types of Melons

- *Canteloupe:* Large round melons with regular indentations. The skin is rough and mottled orange and yellow. The flesh is light orange in colour. From France and Holland. The season is late summer.

- *Charentais:* Small and round with mottled green and yellow skin, the flesh is orange coloured. From France and the season is late summer.

- *Honeydew:* Long oval shaped fruits with dark green skins. The flesh is white with a greenish tinge, imported from Africa and Spain with a season of late summer and into winter.

Nuts include:

Almonds, brazil nuts, chestnuts, cob nuts, filberts, pecans and walnuts.

BEVERAGES

The term beverages on a menu now includes coffees, teas, tisanes, chocolate and other milk drinks (hot and cold) and proprietary drinks such as Bovril or Horlicks.

There is now more choice available. Tea, coffee (in both standard and decaffeinated versions) and a range of other beverages are commonly available throughout the day with a choice of milks, creams (including non-dairy creamers) and sugars (including non-sugar sweeteners). The use of the small coffee cup (demi-tasse) is also on the decline.

Tea

Tea is an evergreen plant and a member of the Camellia family. *Camellia Sinensis* is indigenous to China and parts of India. Left to grow wild the tea plant develops into a tree many metres high, but under cultivation *Camelia Sinensis* is kept to a height of approximately three feet. Today tea is grown in more than 25 countries around the world. The crop benefits from acidic soil, warm climate and where there is at least 130cm of rain per year. It is an annual crop and its flavour, quality and character is affected by the location, altitude, type of soil and the climate.

The lead particle size is referred to as grades. These are Pekoe (pecko)—delicate top leaves, Orange Pekoe—rolled leaf with a slim appearance and Pekoe dust—smallest particle of the leaf size. In between these grades there are a set of grades known as fannings. In tea terminology, 'flush' refers to a picking, which can take place at different times of the year.

Main tea producing countries are:

- **China:** This is the oldest tea growing country and is known for speciality blends such as Keemun, Lapsang Souchong, Oolongs and green tea.

- **East Africa (Kenya, Malawi, Tanzania and Zimbabwe):** This area produces good quality teas, which are bright and colourful and used extensively for blending purposes. Kenya produces bright colourful teas that are easily discernible and which have a reddish or coppery tint, and a brisk flavour.

- **India:** The largest producer of tea. Best known are teas from Assam, strong and full bodied, Darjeeling, delicate and mellow tea and also Nilgiri which is second only to Assam and produces teas similar to those of Sri Lanka.

- **Indonesia:** Teas produced here are light and fragrant with bright colouring when made and are used mainly for blending purposes.

- **Sri Lanka (formerly Ceylon):** Teas here are inclined to have a delicate, light lemon flavour. They are generally regarded as excellent afternoon teas and also lend themselves to being iced.

Service of tea:

Assam: Rich full and malty flavoured tea, suitable for service at breakfast, usually with milk.

Darjeeling: Delicate tea with a light grape flavour known as the 'Champagne of Teas'. Usually served as an afternoon or evening tea with either lemon or a little milk if preferred.

Earl Grey: Blend of Darjeeling and China tea, flavoured with oil of Bergamot. Usually served with lemon or milk.

Iced Tea: A strong tea, which has been cooled and then chilled. It is served with lemon, mint and sugar is offered.

Jasmine: Green (unoxidised) tea, which is dried with Jasmine Blossom and produces a tea with a fragrant and scented flavour.

Kenya: Consistent and refreshing tea usually served with milk.

Lapsang Souchong: Smoky, pungent and perfumed tea, delicate to the palate, which may be said to be an acquired taste. Usually served with lemon.

Russian/Lemon tea: Tea generally made from Indian or Ceylon tea and served with slices of lemon, often in special tea glasses. Sometimes freshly squeezed lemon juice is also offered.

Sri Lanka: Pale golden tea with a good flavour. Ceylon blend is still used as a trade name. Served with lemon or milk.

Tisanes: These are fruit flavoured teas and herbal infusions which are often used for medicinal purposes and are gaining in popularity with trends towards more healthy eating and drinking. Often these do not contain caffeine. Examples are: Herbal teas: camomile, peppermint, rosehip and mint; Fruit flavoured teas: cherry, lemon, blackcurrant, and mandarin orange. These teas are usually made in china pots, or can be made by the cup or glass, and sometimes served with sugar.

Coffee

Coffee beans are grown in many countries in the tropical and sub-tropical belt of South America, African and Asia. Brazil is the world's largest producer, with Columbia second. The trees that produce coffee are of the genus *Coffea*, which belongs to the *Rubiaceae* family. These are the trees *Coffea arabecia* and *Coffea camephora*, usually referred to as *robusta*. Most coffee beans sold as named or branded blends containing a variety of coffees and roastings. There is however a growing trend in featuring beans grown on a single estate.

The beans are roasted to varying degrees to bring out the coffee flavour, the most common degrees of roasting being:

- Light/pale: suitable for mild beans to preserve their delicate aroma
- Medium: gives a stronger flavour and well-defined character

- Full: popular in many Latin countries often producing a bitterish taste
- High: this accentuates much of the strong and bitter aspects of the coffee but can destroy much of the original flavour.

Service of coffee

Americano: Espresso with added hot water to create regular black coffee.

Café Crème: Regular coffee prepared from fresh beans, ground fresh for each cup, resulting in a thick cream coloured mousy head referred to as the crema.

Cafetière: Popular method of making and serving fresh coffee in individual or multi-portion jugs. Often served with hot or cold milk or cream.

Caffé (or Café) Latte: Shot of espresso plus hot milk, with or without foam.

Caffé Mocha (or Mochaccino): Chocolate compound (syrup or powder) followed by a shot of espresso the cup or glass is then filled with freshly steamed milk topped with whipped cream and cocoa powder.

Cappuccino: Espresso coffee topped with steamed frothed milk, often finished with sprinkling of chocolate (powdered or grated).

Decaffeinated: Coffee with caffeine removed. Can be used as an alternative to prepare the service styles listed here.

Espresso: Traditional short strong black coffee.

Espresso Con Panna: Espresso with a dollop of whipped cream on top.

Espresso Doppio: Double espresso served in a larger cup.

Espresso Macchiato: Espresso spotted with a dollop of hot or cold milk or hot milk foam.

Espresso Ristretto: Intense form of espresso, often served with a small glass of ice cold water in Europe.

Filtre (filtre): Traditional method of making coffee. Often served with hot or cold milk or cream.

Iced coffee: Chilled regular coffee sometimes served with milk or simply single espresso topped up with ice cold milk.

Instant coffee: Coffee made from processed powder (often freeze dried). Regular and decaffeinated styles are available.

Jug: Uses a medium to coarse grind. The ground coffee is placed into a jug and boiling water added. After a time the grains will float to the surface. If a spoon is drawn over the surface, the grains will sink to the bottom, but it is still advisable to use a strainer when serving.

Latte Macchiato: Steamed milk spotted with a drop of espresso.

Percolator: Uses a medium grind. A method of making coffee where the ground beans are contained in a filter, which stands in the pot. This method has become less popular because the process boils the coffee as it is being made.

Speciality coffees: These are coffees made in the conventional way to which spirits or liqueurs are added and then double cream floated on top. Sugar is necessary both for taste and to ensure that the cream will float. The main varieties are:

Café Royale—Cognac	*Jamaican/Caribbean*—Rum
Caffé Normand—Calvados	*Monks*—Bénédictine
Caffé Suisse—Kirsch	*Roman*—Galliano
Calypso—Tia Maria	*Rudesheimer*—Asbach brandy
Danish—Gin	*Russian*—Vodka
Gaelic/Highland—Scotch Whisky	*Seville*—Cointreau
Irish—Irish Whiskey	

Note: The names of these speciality coffees and the spirit they contain vary slightly from establishment to establishment.

Turkish/Egyptian: Intense form of coffee made with powdered coffee. This is made from dark roasted coffee in special copper pots. The pots are filled with water, which is then boiled and sugar added. The powdered coffee is then added to produce a very strong beverage. Vanilla pods are sometimes added as flavouring.

Vacuum infusion: Uses a medium grind. This method is characterized by the double pot or glass bowl and filter, which many people know by the trade name 'Cona'—which is the name of the company who made the glass equipment 'Cona'.

COCKTAILS AND MIXED DRINKS LISTING

WHISK(E)Y COCKTAILS

Highball	1 part whiskey Dry ginger ale	Place ice into the highball glass. Add the whiskey and stir to chill well. Add the dry ginger ale to taste. Decorate with a twist of lemon peel.
Highland Cooler	2 parts Scotch whisky 1 teaspoon caster sugar 1 part lemon juice Dashes of Angostura bitters to taste Ginger ale	Shake whisky, lemon juice, sugar and Angostura with ice. Serve in rocks glass with ice and top of with ginger ale.
Manhattan	2 parts American rye whiskey 1 part sweet vermouth	Pour ingredients into mixing glass and stir until well chilled. Strain into a cocktail glass.
	Note: for Dry Manhattan substitute dry vermouth for the sweet.	
Mint Julep	2 parts Bourbon whiskey Soda water to moisten Caster sugar Mint leaves Crushed ice	Place mint leaves and sugar into a highball glass. Moisten with Soda Water and muddle the mixture to dissolve the caster sugar. Add the Bourbon whiskey and fill the highball glass with the crushed ice. Stir and decorate with mint. Serve with straws.
Old Fashioned	2 parts rye whiskey Dash Angostura bitters to taste Caster sugar	In an old-fashioned glass saturate either one lump of sugar, or one heaped teaspoon of caster sugar with Angostura and add a dash of water. Muddle to dissolve caster sugar and then add whiskey. Fill glass with ice, stir and garnish with a slice of orange and a cherry.

Rusty Nail	1 part Scotch whisky 1 part Drambuie	Stir on ice in the bar mixing glass. Always serve on the rocks, with ice partially crushed, in an old-fashioned glass.
Scotch Mist	1 part Scotch whisky Crushed ice Lemon twist Short straws	Fill an old-fashioned glass with crushed ice and pour whisky over ice. Decorate with lemon and add straws (also Bourbon Mist, Rye Mist etc.).
Whiskey Collins	1 part American rye whiskey 2 teaspoons caster sugar 1 part lemon juice Soda water	Collins is a sour served on the rocks in a collins (or highball) glass and topped with soda water. Garnish as a sour but add straws.
Whiskey Fizz	1 part American rye whiskey 1 part fresh lemon juice 2 teaspoons caster sugar Soda syphon	Place the whiskey, fresh lemon juice and caster sugar on ice into the cocktail shaker. Shake well together. Strain into an old-fashioned glass. Garnish with lemon and add straws.
Whiskey Sour	1 part American rye whiskey 2 teaspoons caster sugar 1 part lemon juice	Shake all ingredients well with ice until the caster sugar is dissolved. Strain into a sour (or rocks) glass. Garnish with a slice of orange and a cherry.

Variations are: Gin Sour, Bourbon Sour, Rum Sour (Dark Rum) Scotch Sour, Daiquiri Sour (Light Rum)

GIN COCKTAILS

Claridge	2 parts gin 2 parts dry vermouth 1 part Cointreau 1 part Apricot Brandy	Place all ingredients on ice into a cocktail shaker. Shake vigorously. Strain into a large size cocktail glass. Decorate with a cocktail cherry and a twist of lemon.
Clover Club	2 parts gin ½ part grenadine 1 part fresh lemon juice 1 part white of egg	Place all ingredients on ice into a cocktail shaker. Shake vigorously. Strain into a large size cocktail glass. Decorate with a cocktail cherry and a twist of lemon.

Dry Martini (Gin & French)	2 parts gin ½ part of dry vermouth	Pour the gin and dry vermouth into the bar mixing glass. Stir on ice until well chilled. Strain into a cocktail glass and garnish with either a stoned or stuffed olive on a cocktail stick, or a twist of lemon.
Gibson	2 parts gin 1 part dry vermouth Dash Angostura bitters to taste Dash Orange bitters to taste	Place all ingredients on ice into a cocktail shaker. Shake vigorously. Strain into a cocktail glass. Decorate with a cocktail onion and a twist of lemon.
Gin Fizz	1 part gin 1 part fresh lemon juice 2 teaspoons caster sugar Soda syphon	Place the gin, fresh lemon juice and caster sugar on ice into the cocktail shaker. Shake well together. Strain into an old-fashioned glass. Garnish with a cherry and add straws.

Variations are: Golden Fizz, same as Gin Fizz plus egg yolk; Royal Fizz, same as Gin Fizz plus whole egg and Silver Fizz, same as Gin Fizz plus egg white only

Negroni	1 part gin 1 part sweet vermouth 1 part Campari Dash of soda water	Stir all ingredients over ice in the bar mixing glass. Strain into a collins glass filled with crushed ice. Add the soda water to taste. Garnish with a slice of lemon.
Orange Blossom	1 part gin 1 part fresh orange juice	Shake well with ice and strain into a cocktail glass.
Pink Gin	1 part gin 2 or 3 drops of Angostura bitters to taste Iced water	Place the Angostura bitters into a spirit glass (paris goblet or rocks glass), swill around, and then tip out the excess. Fill the glass with crushed ice and pour over the gin. Serve with iced water according to taste.
Pink Lady	2 parts gin Dash grenadine 2 parts white of egg	Shake all ingredients vigorously on ice and strain into a cocktail glass.

Singapore Sling	1 part gin ½ part Cherry brandy ½ part lemon juice Soda Water	Shake with ice. Serve in a highball glass. Top with soda water and garnish with an orange slice and a cherry.
Sweet Martini (Gin & Italian)	2 parts gin ½ part of sweet vermouth	Method as for dry martini. Garnish with a red maraschino cherry.
Tom Collins	1 part gin 2 teaspoons caster sugar 1 part fresh lemon juice	Shake all ingredients vigorously with ice, and strain into a cocktail glass.
White Lady	2 parts gin 1 part Cointreau 1 part fresh lemon juice	Place all ingredients on ice into a cocktail shaker. Shake well and strain into a cocktail glass. Decorate with a twist of lemon.

BRANDY COCKTAILS

B & B	½ part cognac ½ part Benedictine	Stir well on ice in the bar mixing glass and strain into a liqueur glass (or brandy balloon).
Blue Lady	1 part Blue Curaçao 1 part lemon juice 1 part cognac 1 egg white	Put all ingredients together into a cocktail shaker with ice, shake vigorously and strain into a cocktail glass.
Between The Sheets	1 part cognac 1 part Cointreau 1 part white rum ½ part fresh lemon juice	Shake all ingredients well on ice and strain into an old-fashioned glass.
Brandy Alexander	1 part cognac 1 part single cream 1 part crème de cacao	Shake all ingredients vigorously with ice and strain into a cocktail glass or small brandy balloon.
Sidecar	1 part cognac 1 part Cointreau 1 part fresh lemon juice	Shake all ingredients well on ice and strain into a highball glass partially filled with crushed ice.
Stinger	2 parts cognac ½ part white crème de menthe	Shake ingredients well on ice, until very cold, and then strain into a cocktail glass.

RUM COCKTAILS

Bacardi	1 part Bacardi 1 part fresh lime juice or to taste 1 level teaspoon of caster sugar	Place all ingredients on ice into a cocktail shaker. Shake well. Strain into a cocktail glass. Decorate with a twist of lime peel. Can also be made with grenadine instead of the sugar.
Cuba Libre	1 part white rum 1 part lemon/lime juice Cola to taste	Pour the white rum and lemon/lime juice into a collins glass with ice. Add a slice of fresh lemon/lime. Top up with Cola to taste.
Daiquiri	2 parts Daiquiri white rum 1 part lime juice 1 level teaspoon of caster sugar	Place all ingredients on ice into a cocktail shaker. Shake well. Strain into a cocktail glass and decorate with lemon or lime peel.
Pina Colada	1 part white rum ½ part coconut cream 3 parts pineapple juice 1 dash Angostura bitters	Shake all ingredients vigorously on ice and strain into a collins glass (or Paris goblet). Garnish with fresh pineapple. Add straws.
Shanghai	1 part white rum 1 dash Pernod 1 part fresh lemon juice 2 dashes grenadine	Shake all ingredients well on ice and strain into an old-fashioned glass partially filled with crushed ice.

VODKA COCKTAILS

Black Russian	1 part vodka 1 part Kahlúa	Stir on ice in the bar mixing glass. Serve on the rocks in a cocktail glass.
Bloody Mary	1 part vodka 5 parts tomato juice (or as required)	Place ingredients in the cocktail shaker and shake well on ice. Season and serve in an old-fashioned glass if 'on the rocks', otherwise serve in a collins glass.

Note: To make tomato juice 'spicy' add salt, pepper and Worcestershire sauce. Adding any of the following can also enhance flavour: dash of Tabasco, fresh lemon juice and pepper from the peppermill or cayenne pepper. Garnish can also be varied: stick of celery, carrot stick or a wedge of lemon

Blue Lagoon	2 parts vodka 1 part blue Curaçao Lemonade 1 part double cream	Place the vodka and the blue Curaçao on ice into the cocktail shaker. Shake well. Strain onto crushed ice in a collins glass. Add lemonade and float the double cream on the surface, over the back of a teaspoon.
Harvey Wallbanger	1 part vodka 4 parts or more orange juice ½ part of Galliano	Shake the vodka and orange juice well, on ice, in the cocktail shaker. Strain into a collins glass filled with crushed ice. Float the Galliano on top over the back of a teaspoon.
Moscow Mule	1½ parts vodka 1 part fresh lemon juice Ginger beer to taste	Fill a highball glass with ice. Add the vodka and fresh lemon juice. Stir well to blend and chill. Top with the ginger beer to taste. Decorate with a twist of lemon/lime.
Screwdriver	1 part vodka 4 parts fresh orange juice	Place all ingredients on ice into a cocktail shaker. Shake thoroughly. Strain onto partially crushed ice in a highball glass. Decorate with a slice/twist of fresh orange.
Vodka Martini	2 parts vodka ½ part dry (or sweet) vermouth	Method as for dry martini. Garnish with an olive, twist of lemon peel or a maraschino cherry (name according to vermouth used).

TEQUILA COCKTAILS

Margarita	1 part tequila 1 part fresh lemon juice 1 part Cointreau	Place all ingredients on ice into a cocktail shaker. Shake well. Strain into a cocktail glass rimmed with salt.
Tequila Sunrise	1 part tequila 2 dashes grenadine 4 parts orange juice	Place the tequila and fresh orange juice on ice in a collins glass. Stir well to chill and blend. Add grenadine. Decorate with orange segment or twist of orange peel. Add straws and serve.

WINE BASED COCKTAILS

Kir
1 glass white wine (Dry white Burgundy)
10 to 15ml crème de cassis

Place the crème de cassis in a chilled wine glass. Add the well-chilled white wine. Stir thoroughly.

Mulled wine
2 bottles Burgundy or Rhône red wine
¼ bottle dark rum
½ bottle Dubonnet
½ bottle drinking water
whole orange studded with cloves
2 cinnamon sticks
25g (1oz) sultanas
2 lemon halves
5g (¼oz) mixed spice
1,400g (1lb) jar clear honey

Heat clouted orange for 10 mins in oven to bring out flavour. Tie the mixed spices in a muslin bag to prevent clouding the wine. Place all ingredients except rum into large pot. Hold some of the honey back so as to be able to adjust flavour later. Place pot on low heat and stir occasionally. Bring mixture to boiling point but do not allow to boil. When ready to serve add the rest of the honey to taste and finish with the rum just before serving into small paris goblets. Sprinkle a little grated nutmeg onto the top of each drink.

CHAMPAGNE COCKTAILS

Bellini
2 parts well chilled champagne
1 part fresh peach juice

Prepare in a flute shaped champagne glass by pouring in the fresh peach juice first and topping up with the well-chilled champagne. Garnish with fresh peach.

Black Velvet
Guinness
Chilled dry Champagne

Top up guinness with chilled dry Champagne—often served in silver tankards.

Bucks Fizz
2 parts well chilled champagne
1 part fresh orange juice

Prepare in a flute shaped champagne glass by pouring in the fresh orange juice first and topping up with the well-chilled champagne. Decorate with a curl/twist of orange peel.

Champagne Cocktail	1 Sugar cube Angostura bitters Champagne (well chilled) 1 teaspoon brandy	Place the sugar cube soaked in Angostura into a flute (or tulip) shaped Champagne glass. Pour over the well-chilled Champagne and float the brandy on the surface. Garnish with a slice of orange and a Maraschino cherry.

Note: this cocktail can be made with sparkling wine but should then be called by the name of the wine used and not a Champagne Cocktail

Kir Royale	1 tulip glass dry Champagne 10 to 15ml crème de cassis	Place the crème de cassis in a chilled tulip-shaped glass. Add the well-chilled Champagne. Do not stir.

OTHER COCKTAILS

Americano	1 part Campari ½ part sweet vermouth Soda Water	Place the Campari and sweet vermouth over ice in the bar mixing glass. Stir well to chill and blend and strain into an old-fashioned glass generously loaded with ice. Top up with the soda water to taste. Garnish with a slice of orange.
Cobblers	Sherry or port or brandy, or Champagne etc Fresh fruit pieces	Fill highball/cobbler glass with crushed ice, place fresh fruit pieces into the glass and top up with alcohol. Serve with a straw and spoon (name according to alcohol used).
Coolers	Caster sugar ginger ale Whisky or gin or rum or Cognac or Arrack, etc.	Place ice, two to three teaspoons of sugar and the alcohol, into a shaker and share vigorously. Serve into a highball glass, top up with ginger ale and serve with a straw (name according to alcohol used).

Daisies

Juice of half a lemon
Grenadine to taste
Cherries
Soda water
Whisky or gin or rum or
 Cognac or Peach Brandy
 or Cherry Brandy etc.

Place ice, grenadine and the alcohol, into a shaker and share vigorously. Serve into a Champagne cup, add 3 to 4 cherries and top up with soda water and serve with a straw and a spoon (name according to alcohol used).

Egg-nogs

Cognac or other brandy or
 whisky or gin etc
Whole egg
Nutmeg
Caster sugar to taste

Place ice, whole egg, two teaspoons of sugar and alcohol, into a shaker and share vigorously. Serve into a cocktail glass and sprinkle with grated nutmeg (name according to alcohol used).

Flips

Cognac or Port or Sherry
 or (Rose Flip)
Kirsch and Cherry
Hearing
Egg yolk
1 to 2 teaspoons caster
 sugar to taste
Nutmeg

Place ice cubes, fresh egg yolk, and sugar with 50cl of alcohol into a shaker and shake vigorously. Serve in a cocktail glass with nutmeg sprinkled on the top (name according to alcohol used).

Golden Dream

1 part Galliano
1 part Cointreau
1 part fresh orange juice
1 part single cream

Shake all ingredients vigorously over ice in the cocktail shaker. Strain into a cocktail glass.

Grasshopper

1 part single cream
1 part crème de menthe
1 part white crème de cacao

Place all ingredients over ice in the cocktail shaker. Shake thoroughly. Strain into a cocktail glass.

Grogs

Rum or Arrack or Cognac
 or whisky or gin etc
Half lemon
2 to 3 teaspoons sugar
 according to taste
boiling water

Place 2 to 3 teaspoons of sugar into collins/rocks glass, add alcohol, juice of half a lemon and top up with boiling water. Serve with a tea spoon and garnish with slice of lemon (name according to alcohol used).

Pimms

2 parts Pimms No 1 cup
5 parts or more of
lemonade/tonic water/
Seven-up

Pour Pimms into worthington or highball glass add ice and top up with lemonade or alternatives. Decorate with slice of apple, orange, lemon, lime and a twist of cucumber peal. Alternatively just use mint leaves. Stirrer and straws are optional

Sherry Cup

1 part dry sherry
4 parts Medium cider
Fresh sliced unpeeled
cucumber

Use very chilled ingredients. Put one part of sherry into highball or worthington glass and top up with cider. Garnish with fresh sliced cucumber slices.

NON-ALCOHOLIC COCKTAILS

Fruit Cup

1 part orange juice
1 part grapefruit juice
1 part apple juice
Lemonade/Soda Water

Pour all ingredients, with the exception of the lemonade/soda, onto ice in a glass jug. Stir well to blend and chill. Add sliced fruit garnish. Top up with lemonade or Soda Water. Serve well chilled in highball or worthington glasses.

Pussyfoot

2 parts orange juice
1 part fresh lemon juice
1 part lime cordial
½ part grenadine
1 egg yolk
Soda Water

Place all ingredients with the exception of the soda water on ice into a cocktail shaker. Shake vigorously to blend well together. Strain over crushed ice into a collins glass. Top up with the soda water. Add straws.

Saint Clements

1 part orange juice
1 part Bitter Lemon

Mixed in worthington glass in equal quantities, ice added and garnished with a slice of orange and lemon.

Shirley Temple
/Roy Rogers

ginger ale
Dash of grenadine

Place ice in a highball glass and add a dash of grenadine. Pour over the chilled ginger ale. Decorate with full fruit garnish and add straws.

Note: variations are: ginger ale and fresh lime juice or ginger ale and lime cordial to taste

Tropicana

1 part pineapple juice
1 part orange juice

Mix the well chilled ingredients on crushed ice in a slim jim glass and serve with straws.

GLOSSARY OF SOME CUISINE AND SERVICE TERMS

A

À l'Anglaise	English style
À la broche	Cooked on a spit
Abats	Offal
Aboyer	To bark, shout out the orders
Abricot	Apricot
Aceto	Vinegar (Italian) e.g., Balsamico
Acide	Acid, sharp
Addition	Bill, at the close of the meal
Affiné(e)	Refined, e.g., used at times to describe cheeses
Agneau de lait	Baby lamb wholly milk fed also known as 'agnelet'
Agneau pascal	Spring lamb
Agnelle	Ewe lamb
Aigre	Sour, sharp
Aiguillettes	Long, thin, vertically cut strips of meat from the breast of ducks and other poultry
Ail	Garlic
Aïoli	Garlic mayonnaise from Provençe
Aillé	Flavoured with garlic. *Ailler* to flavour with garlic
Ajo blanco	Purée sauce of garlic and almonds (Spanish)
Al dente	Cooked so as to be slightly firm as for pasta or vegetables
Allumette	Match e.g., as in *Pommes allumette*, matchstick potatoes
Amande	Almond
Amuse-bouche	Small savoury snacks served as a pre-starter in the gift of the house
Amaretti	Macaroons (Italian)
Anchois	Anchovy
Anchoide	Provençal paste of garlic, anchovy and olive oil
Antipasti	Starters (Italian)
A point	Medium rare (steaks)
Arborio rice	Short-fat-grained Italian rice used in the production of risotto

Aroma	Smell, scent or fragrance of food or drink
Aspic	Savoury jelly
Assembly Kitchen	Food production system based on accepting and incorporating the latest technological developments in manufacturing and conservation of food products
Assiette de	Plate of
Au Bleu	Method of cooking trout; when applied to meat it means 'very underdone'
Au four	Baked in the oven
Au gratin	Topped with breadcrumbs and or grated cheese and browned under a salamander (grill)
Au naturel	Uncooked

B

Baba	Polish yeast cake produced from a rich yeast dough often flavoured with rum
Bagel	Type of hard bread roll
Baguette	French bread stick
Bain-marie	Hot water bath or well
Balsamic vinegar	Intense flavoured sweet wine vinegar
Ballotine	Small balls or rolls of meat or poultry. The term is also applied to a boned, stuffed duck
Bard (barder)	To cover or wrap poultry, game or meat with a thin slice of fat bacon so that it does not dry out during roasting
Baron	A saddle of lamb or mutton with the legs attached
Baron de boeuf	Double sirloin
Barquette	Boat shaped tartlet case, filled in a variety of ways
Basil	Herb used for flavouring
Basmati rice	Long grained rice used in Indian cuisine e.g., Biriyani
Bavarois	Bavarian-cream
Beards (ébarber)	To remove the beard from oysters, mussels, etc.
Bearnaise	Warm butter based sauce offered as accompaniment with grilled meats and some fish
Bergamot	An orange scented herb giving a distinctive flavour to Earl Grey Tea. Also used in sweet and savoury dishes
Beignets	Deep fried fritters or doughnuts
Beurre blanc	Light emulsion sauce of white wine, vinegar, finely chopped shallots and butter

Beurre fondue	Melted butter with lemon juice added
Beurre maître d'hôtel	Kneaded butter with lemon juice and chopped parsley added, rolled into a compact cylinder and chilled. Used to garnish some fish, and grilled meat dishes styled 'Vert Pre'
Beurre manié	Butter and flour kneaded together and used to thicken sauces and soups. Literally 'handled butter' or 'kneaded butter'
Beurre noisette	Nut brown butter
Bien cuit	'Well done' term for grilled meats
Blllfold	Style of wallet used for presenting bills and change to the host of a table
Bind (lier)	To thicken soups and sauces with eggs, cream beurre-manié etc; to mix chopped meat, vegetables , etc with sauce
Biriyani	Indicates long grained rice, spiced and coloured yellow with saffron, garnished with hard boiled egg
Bisque	Soup made with various kinds of shellfish
Bistro	Informal style restaurant
Blanc	Water to which flour has been added, used to keep vegetable white, e.g, celery, fennel, artichoke
Blanch	Placing briefly into boiling water or hot fat/oil and then draining and cooling quickly
Blanch (blanchir)	To part cook a food without colouring
Blanquette	White stew usually from veal or lamb
Bleu	Steak very underdone
Bleu, au	Method of cooking freshly killed trout
Blini	Russian small thick savoury buckwheat flour pancake which usually accompanies the service of caviar(e)
Boeuf Bourgignon	Beef casserole made from braising steak flavoured with red wine
Bombe	Iced sweet prepared in a bomb shaped mould.
Bonne bouche	A name given to small savoury dishes and hot hors d' oeuvres
Bordelaise	Rich brown sauce flavoured with red wine
Borlotti	Dry speckled haricot bean
Bortsch	Duck flavoured consommé of East European origins
Bouchée	Small puff pastry patty; a tiny savoury or hors d'oeuvre tit-bit; Bouchées may be filled in a variety of ways
Boudin noir	Black pudding/blood pudding
Bouillabaise	Mediterranean fish style stew flavoured with herbs
Bouillon, court	Liquor for cooking fish
Bouquet garni	Bunch of mixed herbs used for flavouring stocks, stews, sauces and some soups

Braisé	Braised
Braiser	To brown meat, game and poultry or vegetables thoroughly and then finish cooking in a covered vessel with a little liquid or sauce
Braising pan (bisière)	Covered cooking dish
Brasserie	Indicates a small restaurant and bar where food and drinks are served
Breadcrumb (paner)	To cover a piece of meat, fish, poultry etc with breadcrumbs after first dipping it in flour and beaten egg or liquid butter
Brioche	A type of yeast roll
Brochette	Various aliments on a skewer
Brunch	Indicative of a 'late morning meal' that often replaces both breakfast and lunch
Brunoise	Term used to describe cut of tiny dice of vegetables
Bruschetta	Toasted or baked slices of bread, oiled and sprinkled with herbs; often served as an appetiser
Busboy/Girl	American term indicating a person who carries out clearing duties in a food and beverage service area; also used as a general term meaning waiter or server
Butter (beurrer)	To coat or brush the inside of a mould or dish with butter

C

Caffeine	A stimulant found in tea and coffee
Cajun	French American cuisine where the key ingredients used are capsicum, onion, celery, and peppers
Calamari	Squid
Canapé	Small pieces of bread, usually toasted or savoury bases covered with a variety of savoury items, often served as appetisers
Cannelloni	Type of extruded pasta shaped in large rolls, normally filled with cheese or meat and then baked
Canteen	Style of restaurant found in a school, hospital or industrial catering
Cantonese	Form of cuisine, usually found in westernised restaurants and is one of the five main styles of Chinese cuisine
Capon	A chicken with an undrawn weight of 6-9lbs. It is a cock bird fattened for roasting
Caramel	Burnt sugar, commonly known as 'Black Jack'
Caramelise (carameliser)	To line a mould thinly with caramel sugar, or to coat fruit with, or dip it in, crack sugar

Carré	Best end of lamb
Carte du jour	Card/menu of the day
Carte (à la)	Meaning from the card, this is a menu that lists individually priced dishes
Cassata	Layers of different ice-creams, flavoured with liqueur and often containing glace fruits
Casserole	A fireproof earthenware dish or the term for the stew cooked in a casserole dish
Caviar	Roe of the female sturgeon
Célestine	Garnish of fine strips of savoury pancakes (sometimes herbed)
Ceviche	A classic Mexican dish made by marinating or cooking fish or shellfish in a mixture of lime juice and olive oil, tomato, onions and chilli
Chafing dish	Style of frying pan used for cooking at the table
Chapati	Thin unleavened bread
Char grill	Cooking food on a grill which has coke of coals over an 'artificial' electric or gas heat source
Charlotte	Hot or cold sweet with many variations. e.g., Apple Charlotte
Chaudfroid	Sauce for cold buffet work which sets and can then be glazed
Chervil	Herb used in seasoning, also makes an excellent summer soup
Chiffonade	Leaf salads or vegetables cut in very fine shreds sometimes simmered in butter and seasoning
Chilli con carne	Stew of minced meat (usually beef, chillies and red kidney beans
China tea	Green tea (unfermented) usually served with lemon and not milk
Chop suey	Shredded meat cooked with vegetables
Choucroûte	See Sauerkraut—pickled cabbage
Chow mein	Fried noodles with green vegetables and usually meat
Chowder	A creamy soup made from shellfish e.g., Clam Chowder, American in origin
Ciboule	Spring onions
Ciboulette	Chives
Cingalaise (à la)	Curried, with curry sauce
Citron	Lemon
Citron vert	Lime
Citronnat	Candied lemon peel
Citronné(e)	Lemon flavoured
Civot	Applies particularly to 'ragoûts' of furred game especially of hare
Clarify	To clear by removing any impurities e.g, Consommé and many stocks

Clarify (clarifier)	To clear aspic or bouillon by mixing it with egg white beaten with a little water. The liquid is clarified by simmering gently and skimming off impurities as they rise to the top or tapping off the clarified liquid from the base of the pot
Cloche	Dish cover with a handle at the top and used to keep food hot
Coat (napper)	To cover a dish or dessert entirely with a sauce, a jelly, or a cream, to mask, to dip
Cocotte	Small round fireproof dishes for cooking an egg or a ragout, etc, also used to describe a larger oval casserole for cooking chicken etc
Compôte	Fresh or dried fruit cooked in a sugar/fruit syrup—stewed fruit. Also applies to certain dishes featuring partridge and pigeon
Concassé	Rough chopped (tomato) there is also a cooked version with tomato paste and white wine which is used in classical sauces
Condé	Cold sweet made up of poached fruit and a creamy rice e.g., pears
Condiment	A seasoning offered to guests to give added flavour/contrast to a dish served
Confit	Pieces of virtually boneless meat cooked in its own juices and fat: Normally relates to game, duck or goose
Confiture	Jam
Consommé	A crystal clear enriched clarified soup made from beef, poultry, game, fish or vegetable stock. It can be served hot, cold or jellied
Cook-chill	Food production, storage and regeneration method utilising principle of low temperature control to preserve qualities of processed foods
Cook-freeze	food production, storage and regeneration method utilising principle of freezing to control and preserve qualities of processed foods. Requires special processes to assist freezing
Corbeille	Denotes a basket, usually of fresh fruit
Cordial	Usually recognised as a concentrated fruit squash, such as lime cordial
Coriander	Herb or spice with a wonderful warm bitter flavour; used in Asian, Fusion cuisine
Corkage	Charge made for opening and serving bottles brought in by guests
Cos	Lettuce with long, slender and crisp leaves
Coulis	Sauce that may be described as a 'purée of fruit'
Courgettes	Baby marrows

Couronne	The term is used to describe a dish that resembles a crown, e.g., Couronne d'agneau, prepared by placing two raw best ends of lamb back to back and securing them by string. Often prepared with a farce in the centre of the crown. When the joint is cooked it is often garnished with bouquets of vegetables
Court bouillon	Fish stock with white wine or vinegar and a mirepoix
Couscous	Dish of steamed semolina originating in North Africa
Couvent	A cover or place setting; also a guest
Cover charge	An additional charge added to the hosts bill to increase minimum spend
Crème	A term applied to whipped cream, butter and custard creams used to fill or garnish pastries and cakes. It also describes soups, sauces, egg custards, and many sweets. Often dishes are termed à la crème meaning that a quantity of cream has been used in the preparation
Crème anglaise	Rich custard sauce, of pouring consistency, to accompany a sweet
Crème fraîche	Thick cream that has a 'culture' added to it. As a result it has a sharp taste and has become nearly solid
Croissant	Crescent shaped roll, usually made in similar way to puff pastry and sweet to the palate. Often served at breakfast
Croquettes	Minced fowl, game, meat, fish, or vegetables bound with sauce and shaped like a cork. They are usually flour, egg washed and bread crumbed and deep fried
Croustades	Deep, scalloped tartlet cases which may be served with a variety of fillings
Croûtons	Fried bread used as a garnish; for soups they are cut into small cubes, for other dishes in a variety of fancy shapes for e.g., for 'rognons saute turbigo' they are heart shaped with the tips of the heart dipped into the sauce and then chopped parsley
Crudités	Small pieces of crisp raw vegetables with an accompanying savoury dip usually served as an appetiser
Crumb down	To brush debris from the tablecloth between courses, always the main and sweet and between others where viewed necessary
Crustacean	Various types of shellfish
Currie, Kari	A ragoût flavoured with curry spices mainly applicable to lamb, poultry and beef. Curry is derived from the Hindu 'Khura' meaning palatable

Cuisine minceur	Cooking method where lower calorie ingredients are used to replace the traditional rich foods

D

Dahl	Thick puree of lentils offered as an accompanying dish with curry
Dariole	A small beaker shaped mould
Darne	Thick slice through the middle of a round fish, including the central bone, e.g, salmon, cod
Daube	A method of cooking food very slowly in a hermetically sealed dish in order to preserve its full flavour
Délice	Denotes a trimmed and single folded fillet of fish usually sole. More correctly implying/signalling delectability
Demi-glace	Half glaze; A 'mother' sauce frequently used to improve other sauces, soups and stews
Dessert	Traditionally denotes fresh fruit and nuts served from the fruit basket. Today, it can be used to denote the choice of sweets available from the menu
Devilled (à la diable)	Term generally applied to fried or grilled fish or meat prepared with the addition of very hot condiments and sometimes a highly seasoned spiced sauce
Diablotins	Round slices of French bread covered with a thick béchamel sauce flavoured with strong cheese and cayenne pepper sprinkled with fresh Parmesan cheese and gratinated under the salamander (grill). Classically served with vegetable purée soups which are known as Garbure
Dorer	To egg wash (beaten egg mixed with water) (or milk wash) bread, rolls or pastry prior to baking to yield a golden glossy appearance
Du jour	Of the day
Dumb waiter	Another name for the sideboard found in a food service area. Also used to denote the small lift that sends food from the kitchen to the dining room or floors
Duxelles	Mixture of butter, chopped onions, mushrooms, white wine, crumb, seasoning and other ingredients, used for stuffing vegetables and in making sauces

E

Earthenware	Type of strengthened china much used in the hospitality industry
Écrevisse	Crayfish, resembling mini lobsters living entirely in fresh water
Embrocher	To place on a spit for spit roasting or on skewers for grilling or frying
Émince	Finely sliced or shredded. Various sauces can be used to create the dish, e.g., bordelaise, chasseur, piquante, poivrade, Robert, etc
Entrecôte	Literally means between the ribs. Cut between two ribs of beef, e.g., Wing rib. Today a steak cut from a boned sirloin with trimmed fat
Entrée	A meat dish served with a sauce made up of small cuts of meat or poultry. Formerly regarded as an intermediate dish, now more commonly served as the main dish/course
Entremets	Can be used to indicate vegetables and also to indicate the sweet course in the French classical menu (as entremets sucres)
Envoyez	Send. An instruction from the Aboyeur (kitchen caller) to send a dish away
Epigramme	Small fillets of poultry and game, and breast of lamb
Escalope	Thin slice of flattened and boneless veal or beef
Etuver	Method of simmering food very slowly in butter, or very little liquid, in a closed casserole

F

Faites marcher	Begin to send up. An instruction from the Aboyeur (kitchen caller) to get an order he/she will then call out, ready to be sent away
Farce	Savoury stuffing
Fettucine	Thin ribbons of pasta similar to tagliatelle
Filet	Fillet, the undercut of a loin of beef, lamb, mutton, veal, pork and game. Also applies to boned breasts of poultry and boned sides of fish
Filet mignon	Filet from the saddle of lamb. Also indicates a small round fillet steak
Filo pastry	Very thin and crisp paper like pastry which prior to cooking must be kept moist or it will dry out
Fines herbes	Mixed herbs

Flambé	The culinary term flambé meaning to rain spirits on dishes followed by their ignition, providing a controlled pyrotechnical display. Today it has the aim of intensifying flavour and contributing to gastronomic showmanship and odour hedonics
Fleurons	Crescents and other shapes of baked puff pastry used to garnish a variety of dishes
Float	Sum of money of varying denominations placed in the till prior to service commencing
Foie de volaille	Chicken liver
Foie gras	Liver of a specially fattened goose
Four	Baked in the oven
Frappé	To serve an aliment chilled e.g., melon frappé
Friandises	Alternative name for petit fours offered at he end of the meal with coffee
Fricassée	A white stew of chicken, rabbit or veal
Froid	Cold
Fromage	Cheese
Fruits de mer	Mixed seafood
Fumé	Smoked e.g., truite fumé
Fumet	Essence of fish, herbs, game or poultry

G

Galantine	A dish made from poultry or white meat, boned, stuffed and pressed into a symmetrical shape. Served cold, often in chaud froid, glazed with aspic jelly and decorated
Garnish, garniture	Ingredient which decorates, accompanies or completes a dish. Classically, many dishes are identified by the name of their garnish
Gâteau	Sponge cake usually decorated and flavoured or scented
Gazpacho	Cold soup of puréed tomato, cucumber, onion, red pepper, and garlic. Sometimes garnished with croutons
Genoise	Light sponge cake
Gentleman's Relish	Proprietary brand of anchovy paste consumed on hot buttered toasts
Gibier	Term relating to various forms of game
Glace	Ice cream

Glaze (glacer)	To dust a cake or sweet with icing sugar and brown under the salamander. To simmer vegetables, cut into fancy shapes, in butter until they have a glossy coating. To give meat a shiny appearance by frequently basting it. To give cold dishes, cakes and sweets a shiny appearance by coating with aspic or jelly that is on the point of setting
Gluten	Protein substance found in wheat flour
Gnocchi	Classified as a farinaceous (pasta) type dish. There are three types, one based on semolina, one based on choux paste and one potato
Goujons	Thin strips of fillet of fish cooked in various ways. A common method is bread crumbed and deep fried, served with sauce tartare
Goulash	Stew of meat and onions flavoured with paprika
Gratin, au	A dish is described thus when the top has been sprinkled with grated cheese, possibly mixed with bread crumbs and a little butter, and then browned under a hot salamander or in a hot oven
Grissini	Long, thin and crisp bread sticks
Gros sel	Coarse or rock salt
Guacamole	Spicy avocado dip or sauce
Guéridon	The French word guéridon means a round table from which food is processed, carved, completed and served. Guéridon service originated in Russia and was popularised in 19th century France and in early 20th century England
Gumbo	A spicy casserole of seafood and vegetables, which includes okra. In the USA this term applies to many dishes incorporating okra as one of its ingredients

H

Haché	Minced, usually meat
Haggis	Traditional Scottish dish made up from oatmeal and chopped offal, either poached or steamed
Halal	Meat killed and prepared according to Muslim law
Hang	To keep freshly killed meat or game in a cool place for a time so that it becomes more tender
Hash browns	Dish of American origin made up of shredded or purréed potato and onion, bound with egg and fried

Haute cuisine	The highest standard of French cooking and service
Hollandaise	An egg yolk vinegar and butter based sauce. This or one of its derivatives may be offered with grilled fish, steaks etc
Hors d'oeuvres	Preliminary dishes intended to act as appetisers some served hot and some cold

I

Indienne (à l')	Indian style. With rice and curry flavoured sauce

J

Jardinière (à la)	Match stick shape cut of vegetables. Literally 'in the style of the gardener's wife'
Jambon	Ham
Jambonneau	Small ham
Japonaise (à la)	Japanese style.
Jarret	Shin or knuckle
Jugged hare	Hare cooked in a casserole in its own blood and with wine, seasonings and vegetables
Julienne	Style of cut indicating fine, even strips. Attributed to Jean Julien, 18th century chef
Jus	Juice *jus de pamplemousse*—grapefruit juice. *Jus de viande*—gravy
Jus lié	Slightly thickened gravy

K

Kedgeree	Savoury dish of cooked rice, mix with hard boiled egg, smoked fish and may be flavoured with either tumeric or saffron
Kilojoule (kJ)	Metric measure of energy in food
Knead (fraiser)	To work dough on a pastry board or marble slab with the ball of the hand
Kohlrabi	Turnip style vegetable with a swollen, edible stem
Korma	A mild, spicy, meat or poultry casserole that is cooked in a rich coconut sauce
Kosher	Meat killed and food prepared according to Jewish law
Kromeskis	A Polish word having the same meaning as croquette in French

L

Lady's fingers	Another term used to indicate Okra or Gumbo
Lait, au	Denotes 'with milk' as in café au lait
Lard (larder, piquer)	To draw strips of larding bacon through the middle of a piece of meat by means of a larding tube (larder). To lard the surface by means of a larding needle (piquer)
Laitance	The soft roe of a fish. Most notably herring, carp or mackerel are viewed as a delicacy
Lardon	Indicates a strip of bacon or pork fat that may be used to enhance the flavour of raw meat during its cooking process. May also be used as a garnish in both salads and with vegetables
Lasagne	Large flat pieces of pasta. The dish 'lasagne' is made up of layers of lasagne, meat sauce and cheese sauce
Legumé	Vegetable
Lentil	Type of bean, rich in protein and the basic ingredient of dahl
Lié	Thickened or bound. It applies to creams, soups, sauces
Linguini	Pasta cut into long and very thin strips
Longe (loin)	Joint of meat that will include some or all of the ribs
Lumpfish roe	This is the eggs of the lumpfish and is often died black and used as caviar(e)
Lyonnaise (à la)	Denotes a garnish of onions

M

Macaroons	Small, dry, round pastries made of almonds, sugar and the white of eggs.
Macédoine	A mixture of raw or cooked fruits or vegetables which can be served hot or cold. They appear as a small evenly cut dice
Macerate	To pickle briefly, to steep, to macerate or to souse. Generally applied to fruit, usually diced, and then sprinkled with caster sugar and liqueurs in order to improve the flavour
Maître d'hôtel butter	A herb butter containing parsley and lemon. Served with grilled meats and some fish dishes
Mange-tout	A thin, flat green pea. It is eaten whole
Marinade	To soak meat, game etc for a short while to improve flavour and make more tender
Marjoram	Seasoning herb

Marmite, petite	Beef and chicken flavoured clear soup. Also the name given to the container in which the soup is served
Marron	Chestnut
Meat glaze (glace de viande)	Boiled down bone broth of marrow bones etc reduced to a thickness which when cooled turns to a jelly. Used for glazing cooked meats and improving their appearance. Also used to intensify a finished sauce for entrées
Médaillons	'Médaillon' is a general term for any food which is cut into the shape of a medallion. The word also refers to a round, flat slice of meat; a synonym for tournedos of veal, beef and noisette of lamb
Melba toast	Avery thin style of toast
Meunière	Menu term denoting 'shallow fried' e.g., filet de plie menuière
Mignon	A term applied to the tapering end of a whole fillet of beef, a small steak, also to whole fillets taken from lamb, e.g., filet mignon
Minestrone (Italian)	Thick pasta and vegetable soup
Minute steak	Thin tender steak that may be cooked very quickly. Usually batted out fillet steak or sirloin
Mirepoix	A culinary term describing a mixture of roughly cut carrots and onions, and in certain eventualities bacon, bay leaf and thyme. Used to flavour soups, sauces etc
Miroton	Corrupted from Mironton an 18th century dish. A type of stew made from cooked meat, flavoured with onions
Mise en place	The term for all the operations carried out prior to service in the kitchen and restaurant
Morilles	Edible fungus with a delicate flavour
Mornay	Cheese sauce
Moscovite	Muscovite. Of Moscow
Mortadella	Large Italian sausage that has been lightly smoked
Mother Sauce	There are four mother sauces from which many derivates can be produced. They are as follows: demi-glace, velouté, béchamel, and tomato. Mayonnaise and Hollandaise are often added as a mother sauces and derivatives do stem from them
Moule	Mussel, as in moules marinière
Moussaka	Dish of Greek origin. Made up of minced meat and aubergine, with a topping of cheese sauce and baked
Mousse	A light fluffy mixture, which may be sweet or savoury, served hot or cold
Mousseline	Puree strained extra fine and mixed with cream

N

Nappé	To mask or coat evenly with a sauce or jelly
Napolitain	Neapolitan. Of Naples
Nature	Plain boiled
Naturel, au	Plainly cooked food, without additional embellishment or flavouring
Navarin	A brown stew of lamb or mutton with vegetables garnished with button onions and potatoes
Niçoise	French salad dish that traditionally includes green beans, tomatoes, anchovies, olives, and garlic, e.g., salade niçoise
Normand	Norman. Of Normandy
Noisette	Hazel nut. It is also a culinary term for small pieces of meat taken from a loin of lamb, with the bone and the majority of the fat removed. It is also used infrequently to describe small slices of a fillet of veal or beef
Noix de veau	Cushion or nut of veal used for roasting, braising or sauté. Also used for making escalopes and picatta's
Nouilles	Noodles. Prepared from a paste made from flour, eggs, olive oil and salt. Rolled out wafer thin, cut into thin strips and cooked as for other pasta. They are used for garnishing or served as a farinaceous dish.
Nouvelle cuisine	Form of French cooking that promotes healthy foods and lighter saucing to replace very rich dishes of the traditional classic French cuisine

O

Oeuf en cocotte	Egg baked in its own dish, in a baine-marie, in the oven
Oeuf mollet	Soft boiled egg
Oregano	Seasoning herb similar to marjoram
Osso buco (Italian)	Traditionally using slices from the middle of the knuckle of veal resulting in a piece of meat surrounding a piece of bone. Knuckle of veal casserole cooked in a wine, tomato flavoured demi-glace and vegetable sauce. Finely chopped zest of orange chopped garlic and parsley may be used to finish the dish. Traditionally it is served with a risotto scented with saffron
Oyster	A shellfish usually eaten raw

Oyster cruet   This is a set of accompaniments offered with oysters and comprises of cayenne pepper, peppermill, Tabasco sauce and chilli vinegar

P

Paella   Rice dish flavoured and coloured with saffron. Contains chicken, shellfish and various vegetables including peas

Panada   A dough used to bind forcemeat, made from flour, milk or water, eggs and butter.

Panée   A food item floured, egg and bread crumbed and fried

Pannequets   Pancakes. Sweet or savoury. Derived from the the English word for pancakes

Papilotte, en   Cooked in a buttered paper bag or envelope, e.g., fish

Paprika   Powdered red spice used for its flavour and colour in various dishes e.g., Hungarian goulash

Parfait   A light ice which may be prepared from variously flavoured mixtures

Parma ham   Smoked Italian ham

Parmesan   A very hard dry cheese of Italian origin, used in Italian cooking, and usually offered as an accompaniment with pasta dishes

Pasta   Pastes made from wheaten semolina, in a variety of shapes, and dried—Among the best known are macaroni, spaghetti, vermicelli, noodles, and ravioli

Pâté de foie gras   Made by blending together a fine paste of fattened goose livers with finely minced pork and truffles

Pâté maison   A pâté particular to the establishment (house) and made according to the house recipe

Pastillage   Gum paste

Pavlova   A meringue cake filled with cream and topped with fruit

Paysanne   Vegetables cut in small very thin slices

Pêche Melba   A sweet dish made up of peaches, vanilla ice cream and a raspberry sauce (coulis)

Pepperoni   A spicy beef and pork salami

Périgourdin   Of Périgord

Petits fours   The name given to all kinds of very small fancy cakes, crystallised fruits and bon-bons. A variety may be offered with coffee at the conclusion of a meal, sometimes also called friandises

Piémontais   Piedmontese

Pilaff	Rice cooked with meat, poultry, fish etc
Pilau	Indian version of pilaff—Usually includes chicken, mutton, or goat's meat or a mixture of these
Pintade	Guinea fowl
Pintadeau	Young guinea fowl
Pipe	To force a soft mixture or dough through a forcing bag with a plain or fancy nozzle in order to arrange it in a desired pattern or shape
Pipérade	Fluffy omelette with tomatoes, pimento, onions, often served with *Bayonne* ham. Can also be in a scrambled egg form
Pissenlit	Dandelion. Literally 'piss-in-the-bed', stemming from the plants diuretic quality. Also known as *laitue de chien, dent-de-lion and grouin d'âne*
Pluche	Small leaf, especially of parsley or chervil (minus stalks)
Piquante	Pungent, spicy, sharp, appetising. A sharp sauce having demi-glace as its base, to which is added vinegar reduction with crushed peppercorns and chopped shallots and white wine. To complete the sauce, chopped gherkins, parsley, chervil and tarragon are added e.g., sauce piquante
Piqué	Spiked as in *oignon piqué*, peeled onion, with bay leaves attached (pinned) by cloves, used to flavour milk for bread sauce and other preparations
Poché(e)	To simmer dishes in a mould in a bain-marie until done. To cook food in water that is kept just on boiling point (simmering), without actually letting it boil
Poêler	To casserole in butter in a covered dish with no liquid added. The lid is removed shortly before the end to allow the contents to brown. Used only for the better cuts of meat and poultry
Poêlon	A casserole used for pot roasting usually made of earthenware with a lid
Point, à	The degree of cooking of a grilled steak. Denotes medium. Will have a slight pink tinge in the centre
Pois chiches	Chick peas
Poisson(s)	Fish
Poissonier	Fish chef
Poivrade	Peppery. Derives from the French, poivre meaning pepper.
Poivron	Sweet pepper, (green or red)
Polonais	Polish
Pomme de terre	Potato

Popadum	Very fine, thin, and crisp wafer like pancake, made from lentil flour and served with curry
Portugais	Portuguese
Pot roast	This indicates a joint of meat baked in the oven, with stock and vegetables, in a covered pan
Poulet	Chicken
Poussin	Spring or baby chicken
Preserve	In food service this indicates assorted jams that may be offered at either breakfast or afternoon tea
Prix de revient	Cost price
Prix de vente	Sale price
Profiterole	A small choux pastry bun filled with cream and coated in chocolate or other sauce
Profiteroles	Tiny balls of choux paste often filled and used as a garnish for soup but also as a sweet of the same name where they are filled with cream and coated in chocolate or other sauce
Prosciutto	A raw smoked ham that is served sliced very thinly
Provençale (à la)	Cooked with garlic and tomatoes
Pumpernickel	A dark brown or black rye bread. May be used as a base for canapés

Q

Quail	Small game bird
Quenelles	A kind of dumpling made from forcemeat
Quiche	Flan case filled with a savoury egg custard plus other added ingredients, such as vegetables, mushrooms and bacon
Quince	Hard yellow fruit with a delicate scent which when cooked turns pink

R

Rack (of lamb)	Menu term indicating a joint of lamb made up of the best end of lamb, which is usually roasted e.g., carré d'agneau rôti
Ragoût	Casserole of meat, usually lamb or beef
Ramekin	Small circular baking dish holding one portion
Rang	French term indicating the station in a restaurant which may be made up of 20 or so covers
Rare	Underdone degree of cooking of a grilled steak so that the centre is still running with blood

Ratatouille	Vegetable stew flavoured with ground pepper and garlic
Ravigote	A cold sauce comprising vinaigrette, with the addition of finely chopped onions, and capers, flavoured with chervil and tarragon
Ravioli	Very small squares or rounds of nouille paste enclosing a highly flavoured forcemeat
Réchaud	Spirit lamp used for cooking at the table
Réchauffé	A dish often made up of leftovers—a reheated dish
Reduce	To add wine or other liquid to a roux or to pan residue. To boil down to a desired consistency
Régimier	Diet cook
Rémoulade	Mayonnaise containing capers, gherkins, anchovies and herbs for flavouring
Riz à entremets	Sweetened rice
Ris de veau	Calf sweetbreads
Risotto	Savoury rice dish containing vegetables. It is cooked in stock
Roast (rôtir)	To roast
Roe	Fish eggs
Romain	Roman
Roti	A term of Indian origin denoting bread. Usually a flat unleavened bread similar to chapatti
Rôti	On the menu this indicates a roasted item e.g., gigot de porc rôti
Roulade	A stuffed roll of food that may be sweet or savoury i.e., a thin slice of meat stuffed and rolled or a thin flat sponge filled with cream and rolled
Roux	Flour blended with melted butter under heat, used for thickening soups and sauces. It may be white, blond or brown
Royale (à la)	A garnish
Russe	Russian
Rye	Cereal used in the making of bread.

S

Sabayon	Preparation of egg yolks beaten to incorporate air, and used as a basic thickening.
Sablé	shortbread biscuit (variety of)
Saffron	A spice produced from the crocus plant for the flavouring which also colours food bright yellow
Salamander	A grill having top heat, used for cooking and browning
Salami	Italian strongly seasoned sausage, served cold

Salé(e)	Salted, salt. Salted food
Salmis	Game birds and ducks, boned after roasting, placed in a rich sauce and served as a game stew
Salon	Literally 'sitting room', salon de thé—tearoom
Salpicon	Consists of one or more kinds of food, diced small and bound with sauce
Sambal	Condiment that normally contains onion and chillies
Samosa	Small deep fried pastry coated food item with a spicy meat or vegetable filling
Sang	Blood. *Sang cuit*—literally 'cooked blood'
Satay	Cubes of fish or meat on a skewer and grilled over a charcoal grill and served with a thick sauce made from peanuts and lemon juice
Sauerkraut (choucroûte)	Pickled, very finely shredded white cabbage, preserved in brine and fermented with salt, caraway seeds and juniper berries—An national dish of Germany and Alsace, served hot with bacon and sausages
Sauté	To shallow fry to a golden brown colour
Sauter	Quick cooking process to brown quickly in a sauce or frying pan, or toss in fat anything that requires quick cooking at considerable heat
Sauteuse	Shallow pan with slopping sides and a lid, in which food may first be fried and then braised
Savarin	Circular yeast sponge cake, often soaked in rum flavoured sugar syrup and filled with fresh fruit salad e.g., savarin au fruits
Savoyard	Of Savoy
Schnitzel	A term used in Germany and Austria to designate a thin slice of chiefly, veal, but also pork, turkey or chicken usually panéed and pan fried
Selle	Saddle, which comprises two loins undivided
Service cloth	A cloth approximately the size of a table napkin, used by the service staff as a protection against heat and to assist in handling equipment
Shish kebab	Term of Turkish origin indicating small pieces of meat, usually lamb, cooked on a skewer
Shred (émincer)	To cut meat or vegetables into thin slices or strips
Skim (dépouiller)	To remove impurities and fat from the top of soups and broths, being cooked for a long time, by means of a skimming ladle

Smörgasbord	Term of Scandinavian origin which indicates a self service buffet
Smörrebrod	Open sandwich
Sorbet	Soft fruit flavoured water ice, sometimes flavoured with liqueur or wine that may be served as a sweet course of between courses to cleanse the palate
Soubise	Smooth onion pulp served with various meat entrées
Soigne	Handle with special care
Souffle	A very lightly baked or steamed pudding. The description also applies to light savoury creams and to an omelet
Sous-vide	Method of food production, storage and regeneration method utilising principle of sealed vacuum to control and preserve qualities of processed foods. Requires special processes to assist freezing
Soya bean	A round bean similar in size to a pea and rich in protein—also used to make tofu
Soya sauce	A key ingredient of East Asian cuisine made from the soya bean. The Japanese equivalent is 'shoyu'
Spaetzele (spaetzeli)	Swiss and Austrian paste specially made by pressing egg noodle dough through a colander and boiling it in salt water
Spare ribs	The rib bones of beef or pork marinated and then baked or grilled
Spatchcock	Young game bird or chicken that is split open, partially boned and fried or grilled
Spring roll	A dish of Chinese origin, made up of a pancake type roll filled with minced meat and vegetables that is deep fried
Station	When used as a foodservice term this refers to a group of tables/number of covers to be served by specific members of staff
Stillroom	An area in the back of house that provides those items, both food and beverages, not provided by the key sections of the kitchen or the bars
Stillset	Traditional commercial installation consisting of boiler and bulk storage containers for tea, coffee and hot milk
Stir-fry	East Asian process of cooking food which is cooked over a very fast/high heat
Strudel	Fruit sweet made up of either a puff pastry or filo pastry case filled with various mixtures of fruit which may be served hot or cold

Sugar syrup	Sweet liquor of sugar and water boiled together. In cocktail terms this becomes an ingredient for some cocktails and is termed Gomme Syrup
Suprême	Implies the best or most delicate. Denotes the wing and breast of poultry and game. It also applies to a cut of certain fish e.g., salmon
Sweetmeat	Literally means sugar coated confection of some sort of small fancy cakes—also petits fours

T

Tabasco	Pungent Indian pepper sauce, also used extensively in countries with a hot climate, there is also now a milder version
Tandoor	Open topped clay oven
Tandoori	Indicates food that has been cooked in a tandoor
Taramasalata	A dish Greek in origin and made up of fish roe with garlic and olive oil. In appearance it is a pink, creamy paste
Tarragon	A flavouring herb with long, narrow, green leaves
Tartare sauce	A cold sauce with a mayonnaise base, chopped onions, gherkins, capers and chopped parsley, served with deep fried fish
Tartare, steak	Made up of minced raw beef mixed with parsley, capers and finely chopped onion, which is served cold. The mixture is often moulded and a 'well' set in the centre in which is placed a raw egg yolk
T-bone steak	A steak on a 'T'-shaped bone that includes a cut of the fillet and the sirloin of beef
Terrine	An oblong straight sided cooking utensil with a close fitting lid
Timbale	A half conical tin mould of a dish cooked in such a tin
Tofu	Of Japanese origin, it is a highly nutritious curd made from soya beans
Tortilla	Originating in Mexico this is a round, flat pancake made form cornmeal and normally filled with beans or meat and a sauce. Served hot
Tournedos	Fillet steak cut in round, neatly trimmed portions usually pan fried or grilled
Tripe	The lining of a cows stomach
Tronc	The collection of tips received by food service staff, usually distributed on a weekly/monthly basis, on a points system, according to the level and status of job role within the work area

Tronçon	Portion of flat fish cut across the body, e.g., turbot
Truffle	Edible fungus found underground, especially near the roots of oak trees
Truite arc en ciel	Rainbow trout
Truite de mer	Salmon Trout
Truss	To bind or truss poultry or game birds for cooking, to give them a better shape, using a special trussing needle
Tumeric	A mild peppery spice, used in many curry mixtures, called 'haldi' in India
Tureen	A deep covered dish from which soup may be served when working from the guéridon at the guests' table. The tureen may be large enough for one portion or for a number of portions

U

Underliner	An underplate placed underneath another dish or accompaniment

V

Vacherin	A sweet dish made up of meringue and whipped fresh cream
Vanillé	Flavoured with vanilla
Vanille	Vanilla
Vanné	Stirred (sauce) vanner to stir (sauce)
Vapeur	Vapour, water vapour, steam
Varié	Varied, various, miscellaneous
Veau	Veal. Calf's meat
Vegan	A very strict vegetarian
Vegetarian	Someone who does not eat animals or animal products but may sometimes eat fish, eggs and dairy products
Végétarien, -enne	vegetarian
Velours	velvet
Velouté	Velvety smooth rich white sauce made from chicken or fish stock, cream and a blond roux, etc. Also a name given to a certain classification of thick soups with egg yolks and double cream
Venaison	Venison.
Vert cuit	Just sealed, very little cooking undertaken (meat)
Vichysoisse	Thick potato and leek soup, garnished with chives and usually served cold

Vinaigre	Vinegar
Vinaigre de vin	Wine vinegar
Vinaigre d'estragon	Tarragon vinegar
Vinaigré	Flavoured with vinegar
Vinaigrette	Oil and vinegar
Vindaloo	Very hot curry coming from southern India. It is spiced and flavoured with vinegar
Voiture	Term for a trolley used in the food service area e.g., for the service of hors d'oeuvres, sweets, cheeses, liqueurs, and carving
Volailleur	Poulterer
Vol-au-vent	A round or oval case made of puff pastry—A larger edition of a bouchée

W

Waiters friend	Name of a corkscrew and bottle opener combined
Whitebait	Small young fish of the herring family—usually passed through milk and seasoned flour and deep-fried. Eaten whole
Wok	This is a large basin shaped frying pan used in Asian cookery especially for stir-fry dishes

Y

Yaourt	Yoghurt

Z

Zabaglione	This is a light/creamy sweet dish made by whipping together egg yolk, sugar and Marsala over a low heat and is served slightly warm
Zébrine	A striped skin aubergine variety
Zeste	This is the outer skin of citrus peel, without the pith (white part)
Zucchini	Courgette (baby marrow)

ORIGINS OF SOME CLASSICAL MENU TERMS

Classical menu terminology is a *meta language*. It has been influenced by many factors and the naming of dishes in the classical répertoire allows precise interpretation by the chef, gourmet, gastronome and any other individuals who are interested in the art and science of cuisine. The terms used in *Le Répertoire de la Cuisine* still represent the international language of European cuisine for hospitality businesses.

AFTER RESTAURANTS

D'Antin   Paris restaurant, which gives its name to a poached turbot dish similar to Dugléré but garnished with croûtons fried in butter.

Delmonico   Renowned New York restaurant which gives its name to a method of preparing potatoes and a salad.

Maxim   This well-known Parisian restaurant has an egg dish named after it

Café Riche (Paris) Method for preparation of fish, especially sole, and name for a sauce, it also describes a method of garnishing small cuts of meat.

Voisin (Paris)   Gives its name to a potato dish. Similar to Pommes Anna.

AFTER RESTAURATEURS

Louis Bignon   Celebrated 19th century Paris restaurateur with an egg dish named after him.

Marguéry	Paris restaurateur (1834–1910), and creator of a sole dish carrying his name.

AFTER CHEFS

Antoine Beauvilliers	(1753–1817) Opened one of the first restaurants in Paris in the 1780s and was author of L'Art du cuisinier. A garnish for large joints of braised meats is named after him.
Marie Antoine Carême	Celebrated chef and author of several books (1783–1833). Among dishes he created that bear his name are Perdreau Carême and Bécasse Carême.
Pièrre Cubat	Chef to Emperor Alexander II of Russia. A method of preparing fish bears his name.
Dugléré	(1805–1884) Chef at the Café Anglais. Methods of preparing sole and turbot are named after him.
Auguste Escoffier	Author and celebrated chef (1846–1935). Most of Escoffier's dishes were named for other people, for example Nellie Melba and Sarah Bernhardt. However, several sauces and a cold dish bear his name.
Jean Julien	The term julienne describes a method of cutting vegetables into very fine strips. (Circa 1700s).
Lagupière	Chef to Napoleon and Prince Murat. A sauce and two fish dishes take the name. A feature of these dishes is truffle. Carême also dedicated many dishes to Lagupière.
Vatel	Worked for Louis XIV of France (reputed to have taken his own life because a fish course for a special banquet was not ready on time). A fish dish was created in his name.

AFTER GOURMETS / GASTRONOMES

Baron Brisse
Writer and gastronome (1813–1876) whose name describes a preparation for red mullet, sole fillets and a garnish for small cuts of meat.

Joseph Berchoux
A consommé and a pheasant dish are named after this gourmet (1768–1835). He was also a poet and wrote a poem titled Gastronomie. A feature of dishes named after him, is game.

Brilat-Savarin
Gastronome, magistrate, politician and author of *Physiologie du gout* (1755–1826). Jean-Julien created an enriched yeast cake which eventually had the 'Brillat' part of the name dropped and is today better known as 'Savarin'. Marie Antoine Carême also created a salmon dish, an omelette and a garnish in his name.

Jean Jacques Cambacères
High Chancellor of the French Empire appointed by Bonaparte, he was later made Duke of Parma. Also renowned gourmet with a method of preparing salmon trout and a cream soup with pigeon and crayfish named after him. (1754–1824).

Viscount François Chateaubriand / Châteaubriant
Gourmet and French Ambassador to England (1768–1848). His chef, Montmireil, created a method of preparing the head of beef fillet (thickest part) in his honour.

Lucus Licinius Lucullus
Wealthy Roman General and gastronome renowned for his luxurious banquets. Several dishes carry the name Lucullus, most requiring elaborate preparation and costly ingredients.

Charles Monselet
French gastronome and author of assorted gastronomic works, the best known of which was *Almanach des gourmands* (1825–1888). Many dishes are named after him with the distinctive feature of

globe artichokes, and truffles with potatoes fried in butter.

AFTER ROYALTY

Albert, Prince Consort
Francatelli, Queen Victoria's chef created a sauce and a pudding and dedicated them to Albert.

Princess Alice Countess of Athlone
Sister of King Edward VII of Great Britain. Auguste Escoffier created a method of preparing sole and a sweet in honour of Princess Alice.

Queen Alexandra
Wife of King Edward VII of Great Britain. Many dishes bear the name Alexandra. Both Escoffier and Ménager created dishes, which include one for tournedos, a sole dish, chicken dishes, and two sweet dishes. A key feature of the savoury dishes is the inclusion of points of asparagus.

Louis Charles Philippe Nemours
The Duke de Nemours, 2nd son of Louis Philippe King of France. (1814–1896). A garnish and other dishes are named after him.

Henry IV
King Henry IV of France (1553–1610). He married Marie de Médicis, and she continued to influence him through her Italian cooks at the Court. Several dishes are named after him. A common characteristic of them is sauce béarnaise.

Impératrice (à la)
Literally, 'empress style'. A chicken dish was created/styled in honour of the Empress Marie Louisse. A rice dish Riz Impératrice (condé with candied fruits) was reputedly inspired by the Empress Eugénie.

Marie Louise
Empress of France (1791–1847). The 2nd wife of Napoleon I. There are many dishes named in her honour, the most well known are a chicken dish, a sole dish and a bombe.

Victoria	Queen of Great Britain, and from 1876 Empress of India. (1819–1901). Her chef Francatelli dedicated many dishes in her honour.

AFTER MISTRESSES

Agnès Sorel	Mistress to King Charles VII of France from (1444–1450). She was also known as 'Dame de Beaute'. During his protracted dalliance it is thought his interest in his country's affairs were due largely to Agnès Sorel. Taillevent, Charles VII chef, created a soup, an omelette, a chicken dish, and a method of preparing veal. A feature of all of these dishes, which were adapted by Escoffier, is the inclusion of mushrooms.
Belle Gabrielle	Gabrielle d' Estrées mistress to King Henry IV of France. La Varenne (circa 1600s), Henry's chef, created a consommé and a chicken sauté.
Dubarry	Comtesse du Barry (1746–1793). Mistress to Louis XV. The title Dubarry signifies that cauliflower features prominently or is used as part of the garnish. Comtesse du Barry is said to have styled her hair in a fashion reputed to have resembled that of a cauliflower.
Lavallière	Louise Françoise de la Vallière (1644–1710). Official mistress of Louis XIV. A garnish applied to poultry and sweetbreads, an egg dish, a soup and a sole dish are named after her. Lavallière garnish (for chickens and sweetbreads) includes truffles à la serviette, lambs sweetbreads and crayfishes.
Montespan	Françoise Athénais de Pardaillan, Maquise de Montespan (1641–1707). She became mistress to Louis XIV in 1667, with whom she had seven children. A soup and a sole dish are named after her.

Pompadour	Jeanne Antoinette, Marquise de Pompadour (1721–1764). A renowned courtesan of the reign of Louis XV. Madame de Pompadour was a political player and made herself indispensable to Louis. Many dishes are styled 'Pompadour', most of which feature truffles.

AFTER NOBILITY

Doria	The family name of an ancient and noble Genoese family. Many (19th Century) dishes carry this name and a characteristic feature of them is the inclusion of cucumber as a prominent aliment.
Marie Walewska	A Polish Countess (1789–1817). Mistress of Napoleon Bonaparte, with whom she had a son. A poached fish garnish is named in her honour.
Arthur Wellesley Wellington	First Duke of Wellington (1769–1852). A famous English General who defeated Napoleon I at Waterloo (1815) Filet de boeuf Wellington was named in his honour.

AFTER PROMINENT INDIVIDUALS

Aiglon	Based upon a nickname (Eagle) given to the son of Napoleon I and Marie Louise of Austria. Laguipière created a fish dish and an iced bombe and another sweet which are all known by this name.
Cyrano de Bergerac	A consommé and a garnish for cutlets were created by Jules Hépy, chef of the Grand Café de la Paix. This was done in honour of the hero of Edmond Rostand's play, Cyrano de Bergerac.
Guiseppe Garibaldi	19th Century Italian patriot after whom a consommé and a type of biscuit is named.

Stanley	A Welsh explorer of Africa (1841–1904). Famed for his relief of David Livingstone, but more than this for his discovery and development of the Congo. The main feature of dishes bearing his name is the use of curry powder.
Antoine Augustin Parmentier	Writer, economist and agronomist (1737–1813) who popularised the use of potatoes as a food. He invented many ways of cooking potatoes. The appearance on a menu of the designation Parmentier will indicate the presence of potatoes in the dish.
Pojarski	(1578–1642) Russian Patriot, head of the anti Polish movement. A veal preparation takes his name.
Pièrre de Villeneuve	A French Admiral who commanded the French fleet at the battle of Trafalgar (1805). A venison dish and a consommé are named after him.

AFTER SAINTS

Saint Antoine	Saint Anthony. Patron saint of swineherds. Some pork dishes take on this name.
Saint Hubert	The patron saint of hunters. He has dishes relating to game and those flavoured with game named after him.
Saint Honoré	Bishop of Amiens circa A.D. 660. Saint Honoré is the patron saint of pastry cooks and bakers. A famous and elaborate gâteau is named after him.
Saint Jacques	Saint James. A variety of table grape and also short for *coquille Saint Jacques*—scallop.
Saint Francis Xavier	Xavier was a Jesuit missionary. A consommé and a velouté soup are named after him.

Saint Martin
Bishop of Tours and Roman legionary—Saint Martin le Beau in Touraine is renowned for fine table ducks. *Caneton Saint Martin.*

Saint Pierre
Saint Peter. John Dory, a spiny fierce looking fish with a large mouth and dark spots on each side of its back are said to be the thumb prints of Saint Peter.

Saint Sylvestre
In many parts of Europe Sylvestre is celebrated—New Years Eve.

AFTER COUNTRY OF ORIGIN

Africaine (à l')
African style, featuring tomatoes, aubergines, flap mushrooms cooked in oil.

Algérienne (à l')
Allied with Algeria. Often the name of a garnish applied most especially to large pieces of meat, consisting of small tomatoes cooked in oil and sweet potato croquettes, or sweet potatoes cooked in butter.

Allemande (à l')
German character. Applies to dishes prepared in a particular manner peculiar to Germany. A dish garnished with sauerkraut and pork, or dishes featuring smoked sausages, noodles tossed in butter and mashed potatoes can all be styles à l'Allemande.

Américaine (à l')
Used for various fish, meat eggs and vegetable preparations which usually include tomatoes, bacon and red peppers. One of the most known is *Homard à l'Américaine.*

Anglaise (à l')
English style. Usually implies a plain style either boiled in water or roasted.

Égyptienne (à la)
Egypt. Purée égyptienne features yellow split peas.

Française (à la)   French style or French in origin. It is used to describe many quite simple preparations as well as the more elaborate. Both method of cooking and garnish various too frequently to be too prescriptive here.

AFTER GASTRO-GEOGRAPHIC REGIONS

Alsacienne (à l')   French Province of Alsace. Dishes with this designation usually feature specialities of the area such as foie gras, ham, sauerkraut and sausages as the predominating ingredient.

Andalouse (à l')   Andalusian style. Characterised primarily by tomatoes, pimentoes, aubergines, and rice pilaff. Sauce andalouse is a mayonnaise flavoured with tomato garnished with tiny dice of sweet pimento.

Argenteuil (à l')   A district in France celebrated for its asparagus, an example of its use appears in 'potage Argenteuil'. The name when used frequently implies that asparagus will feature prominently in the dish.

Badoise   From the German town of Baden. There are two garnishes served with dishes of this name. One is served with large joints of meat and features braised red cabbage, lean bacon and mashed potatoes. The second is for smaller cuts, tournedos and noisettes, and features stoned cherries.

Dauphinoise (à la)   Dauphine region of France. Most associated with potatoes. Gratin dishes of many kinds (potatoes, macaroni, crayfish tails, meat) are popularised here.

Dieppoise (à la)   The French port of Dieppe. The port is noted for its shrimps. The classical fish dish 'Delice de sole Dieppoise' features shrimps, mussels and white mushrooms, and white wine sauce.

Niçoise (à la)	From Nice, on the French Riviera. The main characteristic of dishes here is that tomatoes come as standard. Oil and garlic also feature in many of the dishes.

AFTER COMPOSERS OR WORKS

Aïda	Aïda is a famous opera composed by Guiseppe Verdi (1813–1901). Casimir-Moisson, a celebrated chef at the Maison-Dorée patronised by Verdi, named Aïda in honour of Verdi. Turbot Aïda, a soufflé, a bombe and a mixed salad carry the name.
François Adrien Boïeldieu	A French Composer. Between 1804 and 1810 Boïldieu was Chapel-Master and Director of the Opera in St Petersburg. The developer of comic opera into an early form of romantic opera. Dishes believed to have been created by Carême are named after him and include a consommé, a sole dish and a methode of preparing poularde.
Alexander Etienne Choron	A French musician who composed several overtures (1772–1834). Director of the Paris Opera. Choron also applies to a sauce, a garnish and a method of preparing noisettes.
Jules Massenet	A French Composer (1842–1912). Composed comic operas. His name applies to egg dishes and a garnish for small cuts of meat. Potatoes Anna and artichoke bottoms feature.
Giacomo Meyerbeer	A famous German Composer (1791–1864). An egg dish carries his name.
Wolfgang Mozart	A famous Austrian Composer (1756–1791). Vincent La Chapelle produced a garnish for entrées in his honour.

This comprises: Artichoke bottoms, filled with celery purée, copeaux potatoes (potatoes cut in ribbons, fried in deep fat and served very dry).

Gioachino Antonio Rossini	A famous Italian operatic Composer (1792–1868). Musical director of the Théatre Italien in Paris in 1824. Rossini is associated with numerous dishes, of which a common feature is foie gras and truffles. Rossini was reputed to have been most partial to both. Rossini is credited with the invention of Tournedos Rossini.
Sir Arthur Seymour Sullivan	An English Composer of comic opera (1842–1900). Escoffier dedicated a sole dish for him at the Savoy Hotel.
Guiseppe Fortunino Verdi	An Italian Composer (1813–1910). His most popular operas were Rigoletto (1851) Il Trovatore (1853) and La Traviata (1853). Several dishes are named after him including one for tournedos.

GENERAL ORIGINS

Aiguillette	Literally 'little needle', *aiguille* being French for needle. A long thin slice of choicest and most tender meat taken from either side of the breastbone of a duck or other fowl.
Bouchée	Literally, 'mouthful', comprise small light pastry or vol-au-vents filled with an array of savoury mixtures. Bouchées were often created by Louis XV's gourmet queen, 'Marie Leszcinska'.
Caesar Salad	Invented in 1924 by Caesar Cardini, who operated a restaurant in Tijuana, in northern Mexico. It is today an international institution, most prized by American's. Tradition also holds that the dressing is flamboyantly prepared at the table. Chicken

Caesar (with sliced chicken breast) is a more modern addition to the original.

Canapés

Originate from 'Zakouska's' (Russian in origin) meaning snack. Served about one hour in advance of dinner when guests would be called to an adjoining hall or parlour to the dining room. Eventually they were introduced to Europe (1800s) where these tit-bits would be consumed in the lounge area where guests sat upon sofas, which in that period in France were known as 'Canapes'. Hence through the passage of time the appellation entered the language of cuisine in preference to the term Zakouska.

Cappuccino

Establishing itself in English coffee bars of the 1950s. An Italian coffee term and one of the mainstays of Italian coffee culture. A combination of real espresso smoothed out with both steamed and frothed milk creating a luxuriant cap said to resemble the hooded robe worn by the monks of the Order of Minor Capuchins, an independent branch of Franciscans. Derived from the Latin *cappa* 'hood' which comes from *caput* 'head'.

Carbonnade

Has the literal meaning 'glowing coals' *(charbons ardents)* indicating not simply grilling over charcoal, but also braising in the fire. *Carbonnade de boeuf à la flamande* is braised beef and onions flavoured with beer and herbs. *Carbonnade nîmoise* comprises lamb or mutton baked with potatoes, herbs and garlic.

Carbonara

The suggested origin comes from members of the Carbonari, a 19th century secret society working for a unified Italy. They got the name for they disguised themselves as *carbonari*, 'charcoal burners' after being driven deep into the forest of the Abruzzi. In Italy it is a dish of spaghetti or other pasta with the appellation *alla carbonara* having a sauce produced from eggs, onion, olive oil, cream and strips of bacon.

Cardinal (à la)   Literally: 'cardinal's style'. Having the colour pink or red after the cardinal's habit. Often referred specifically to Cardinal Mazarin. *Homard Cardinal*, comprises lobster with Cardinal sauce glazed under the salamander. *Sauce Cardinal* is a lobster sauce with truffles and diced lobster.

Carpaccio   Named in honour of the Italian painter Vittore Carpaccio (c.1460–c.1525). Italian antipasto. Raw beef fillet sliced wafer thin. Served often with olive oil, lemon and shaved parmesan cheese. Originated on the occasion of an exhibition of Carpaccio's works in Venice in 1963.

Carpet-bag steak   The term first recorded in 1958. A preparation for a piece of rump steak. A slit is cut in the steak and oysters are stuffed into it. The steak is then baked. Mainly an Australian preparation.

Ciabatta   Literally, 'slipper' because of its vaguely shoe like shape. It is obtained via Turkish, of Persian *ciabat*. Ciabatta is a type of Italian loaf produced from dough loaded with olive oil.

Clamart   A garnish which consistently highlights fresh peas. Stemming from a locality near to Paris renowned for its market produce.

Coffee   The origin of coffee is shrouded in the myths of the Middle East. One story has it that the goats' of a young goatherd, Kaldi, did not return from grazing one night. The next morning he went looking and found them dancing around a cluster of dark leaved trees with red berries. He tasted the berries and was soon dancing with his goats. He is said to have mentioned the experience to some monks from a nearby monastery and one of them tried and soon neither he nor the monks had problems staying awake at prayers! The news of the wakeful monastery spread and the success of the berries was assured.

Coquille Saint-Jacques

Scallop. Also known as *'peigne'*, *'pélerine'*. Literally, 'pilgrim'. Also *godfiche*. The scallop is a shellfish with white flesh and orange coral. The shell was the badge of the pilgrims to the shrine of Saint James (Saint Jacques) in Spain.

Crêpes Suzette

Originating around the turn of the 20th century, precise origins are not clear. The chef Henri Charpentier cites his originating of the dish at the Café de Paris, Monte Carlo in 1896 for the Prince of Wales, naming it in honour of the Prince's companion on that occasion. This however has been proven inaccurate. Escoffier makes first reference to the crêpes in print in his book Modern Cookery (1907) referring to them by the English name of Suzette pancakes. Crêpes Suzette were at one point the epitome of luxurious dessert dining, featuring in all of the very best hotels and ocean liners as can be seen from the statement: 'crêpes Suzette are pancakes raised by Cunard to a remarkable point of perfection (Vanity Fair, **9** 1928).

Croque-Monsieur ou Madame

Literally 'crunch-sir' or 'munch-sir' *croquer* being French for 'crunch'. It is basically a cheese and ham toasted sandwich first seen around the turn of the 20th century legend having it that it was first produced under that appellation in a café on the Boulevard des Capucines in Paris. More recently it has been served topped with a fried egg and takes the designation *croque madame*.

Egyptiène (à la)   Deriving from Egypt. The soup, *'purée Egyptienne'* is prepared from yellow split peas.

Fermière (à la)   Farmers style, features the inclusion of vegetables as garnish. For example, carrots, onions, turnips and celery. It is cut mainly in paysanne, and is used with large joints of meat and poultry.

Florentine (à la)   Derives from Florence, where Italian cooks popularized the inclusion of spinach in France. The term Florentine applies to numerous egg, fish, meat and poultry garnishes all featuring spinach.

Langues de chat   Literally 'cat's tongues'. They are small tea or dessert biscuits. The term is to a lesser extent used in describing the finest wafers of chocolate.

Lobster Newburg   The recipe for this dish was brought to the world famous Delmonico's restaurant in Lower Manhattan opened in 1831. It is a restaurant that revolutionised public dining in America. The recipe was given over by Ben Wenberg, a sea captain and regular diner. Charles Delmonico being so delighted with the dish, named it Lobster à la Wenberg. Through time Wenberg and Delmonico had a falling out and, in anger, Delmonico renamed the dish Newberg by reversing the first and third letters. Through time Newberg changed through mispronunciation and spelling to Newburg and the name is used in this format throughout the world today.

Restaurant   *'Venite ad me omnes qui stomacho laboratis et ego restaurabo vos'* (come to me, all whose stomachs labour and I will restore you). The above literary joke in culinary Latin was inscribed on a sign above a bouillon maker, or soup-vendor's establishment in Rue Bailleul in Paris. Chefs and gastronomes remember the inscription because the premises were to become the first ever to be recognised as a restaurant.

Tea

Discovered more than 5,000 years ago by the Chinese Emperor, Sheng Nung. One legend says that whilst travelling around his empire he sheltered under a tree to boil his drinking water and a leaf from the tree, a *Camellia Sinensis*, fell into his boiling pot of water resulting in the first brew of tea.

Vichysoisse

Although it has a French name this American soup was created by Louis Diat chef at the Ritz Carlton Hotel in 1910. The soup is based on leeks or scallions, potatoes and double cream and is served very well chilled, it must also be thick and very creamy.

VOCABULARY

French	English	German
A		
abricot	apricot	Aprikose
absinthe	wormwood	Wermut
acide	acid	sauer
addition	bill	Rechnung
adoucir	sweeten (to)	versüßen
agiter	shake (to)	Schütteln
agneau	lamb	Lamm
agneau de lait	spring lamb	Milchlamm
aiglefin	haddock	Schellfisch
aigre	sour	sauer
aiguille	larding pin	Spicknadel
aiguillettes	slices	Scheiben
ail	garlic	Knoblauch
aile	wing	Flügel
aile de poulet	wing of chicken	Hühnerflügel
airelle rouge	cranberry	Preißelbeere
aliment	food	Nahrung
allumettes	matches	Zündhölzer
alose	shad	Maifisch
alouette	lark	Lerche
aloyau	sirloin	Rindsrükenstück
alsacienne	Alsatian style	Elsäasseerart
amandes	almonds	Mandeln
amidon	starch	Stärkemehl
amourette	marrow	Mark
ananas	pineapple	Ananas
anchois	anchovy	Sardelle
aneth	dill	Dill
angélique	angelica	Engelwurz
anguille	eel	Aal
apre	herb, sharp	herb, scharf
arête	fishbone	Gräte

French	English	German
aromatique	aromatic	duftig
arôme	aroma, flavour	Duft
artichaut	artichoke	Artischocke
asperges	asparagus	Spargel
assiette	plate	Teller
assortiment	selection, assortment	Auswahl
aubergine	eggplant, aubergine	Eierfrucht, Aubergine
avoine	oats	Hafer

B

French	English	German
baies	berries	Beeren
baie de genièvre	juniper berry	wacholderbeere
bar	bass	Barsch
barbeau	barbel	Barbe
barbue	brill	Butt
basilic	sweet basil	Basilikum
baudroie	monkfish	Angler
baveuse	soft	Weichgebacken
bécasse	woodcock	Waldschnepfe
bécassine	snipe	Sumpfschnepfe
beignets	fritters	Krapfen
beignets de pommes	apple fritters	Apfelküchlein
betterave	beetroot	Rote Beete
beurre	butter	Butter
beurre clarifié	melted butter	Geklärte Butter
beurre fondue	clarified butter	flüsige Butter
beurre manié	kneaded butter (with flour)	Mehlbutter
bien cuit	well-done	durchgebraten
bière	beer	Bier
bière anglaise	ale	englisches Bier
bière blanche	wheat beer	Weißbier
bière de garde	lager	Lagerbier
bigarade	bigarade	Pomeranze
biscotte	rusk	Zwieback
biscuits au fromage	cheese biscuits	Käsebiskuits, Kaiserschöberln

French	English	German
blanc d'oeuf	white of egg	Eiweiß
blanchir	make white, blanch (to)	Weiß machen
blanquette de veau	stewed veal in white sauce	Weiß Kalbsragout in weißer sauce
blé	corn	Korn
boeuf	beef	Rindfleisch
boeuf braisé	braised beef	Schmorbraten
boisson	drink	Getränk
bolet	mushroom (type of)	Steinpilz
bombe glacée	ice-bomb	Eisbombe
bondelle	silver trout	Silberforelle
bordelaise	Bordelese style Bordeaux style	Bordeleserart
bouchon	cork	Korken
boudin	black pudding	Blutwurst
bouilli	boiled	Gesotten, gekocht
bouillon	beef broth	Fleischbrühe
boules	balls	Kugeln
bourgeoise	bourgeois style	Bürgerliche Art
bouteille	bottle	Flasche
boyau	intestines	Darm
braisé	braised, stewed	geschmort
brème	bream	Blei, Brachse
brochette	skewer	Spieß
brochet	pike	Hecht
broyer	rub, pound (to)	reiben, drücken
brûler	burn (to)	verbrennen
buffet froid	cold buffet	Kaltes buffet, kaltes Büffet

C

French	English	German
cabi, chevreau	kid	Zicklein, Kitz
cabillaud	cod	Kabeljau
cacao	cocoa	Kakao
café	coffee	Kaffee
cafetière	coffee pot	Kaffeekanne
caille	quail	Wachtel
camomille	camomile	Kamille

French	English	German
canard	duck	Ente
canard sauvage	wild duck	Wildente
caneton	duckling	Junge Ente
cannelle	cinnamon	Zimt
carafe	carafe, decanter	Karaffe
carbonade de boeuf	beef carbonade	Rindfleischkarbonade
carcasse	carcase	Gerippe
cardamome	cardamom	kardamom
cardon	cardoon	Kardone
carotte	carrot	Karotte, Möhre
carpe	carp	Karpfen
carré d'agneau	best-end of lamb	Lammrippenstück
carré de mouton	best end/loin of mutton	Hammelkarree
carte des mets	menu card	Speisekarte
carte des vins	wine list	Weinkarte
cassis	blackcurrant	schwarze Johannisbeere
cassonade	moist brown sugar	brauner Zucker
catalane	Catalonian style	Katalanische Art
cave	cellar	Keller
caviste	cellar man	Kellermeister
caviar	caviar(e)	Kaviar
cayenne, poivre de	cayenne pepper	roter Pfeffer
céleri	celery	Sellerie
céleri-rave	celery root	Knollensellerie
cendre	ashes	Asche
cèpe	mushroom (type of)	Steinpilz
cerf	deer	Hirsch
cerfeuil	chervil	Kerbel
cerise	cherry	Kirsche
cervelle	brain	Hirn
chalumeau	straw	Trinkhalm
champignon	mushroom	Champignon
chamois	chamois, goat	Gemse
chandelle	candle	Kerze
chantrelle	egg mushroom	Eierschwamm
chapelure	breadcrumbs	Brotkrümel
chapon	capon	Kapaun

French	English	German
châtaigne	chestnut	Kastanie
château	castle, large house	Schloß,
chaud	hot	heiß
chaudière	steam kettle	Dampfkessel
chef de cuisine	head of the kitchen	Küchenchef
chèvre	goat	Ziege
chevreuil	venison, deer	Reh
chicorée	endive	Endivie
chocolat	chocolate	Schokolade
choix	choice	Wahl, Auswahl
chou	cabbage	Kohl
chou-fleur	cauliflower	Blumenkohl
choucroute	sauerkraut	Sauerkraut
choux de bruxelles	Brussels sprouts	Brüsseler Kohl, Rosenkohl
ciboulette	chives	Schnittlauch
cidre	cider	Obstler, Apfelwein
cigogne	stork	Storch
citron	lemon	Zitrone
clair	clear	hell, klar
clarifier	clear, clarify (to)	klären, Läutern
clou de girofle	clove	Gëwurznelke
clovisse	clam	Muschel
coshon, porc	pork	Schwein
cochon de lait	suckling pig	Spanferkel
coing	quince	Quitte
colin	hake	Seehecht
compote	stewed fruit	Kompott
concasser	crush, pound (to)	Zerstoßen, Stampfen
concombre	cucumber	Salatgurke
condenser	condense (to)	eindicken
condiment	seasoning	Gewürz
confiserie	confectionery	Konditorei
confiseur	confectioner	Konditor
confiture	jam	Konfitüre
consommé	clarified soup	Kraftbrühe
consommé de volaille	clarified chicken soup	Geflügelkrafbrühe
contrefilet	sirloin (of beef)	Lende

French	English	German
coq	cock	Hahn
coq de bruyère	grouse	Auerhahn
coquetier	egg cup	Eierbecher
coquillage	shellfish	Muscheltiere
coquille	shell	Schale
corail	coral	Koralle
corbeille	basket	Korb
cordon	thread, ribbon	Schnur, Band
coriandre	corainder	Koriander
cornichon	gherkin	Essiggurke
côte de veau	veal cutlet	Kalbsrippe
côte de porc	pork cutlet	Schweinskotelett
côtelette	cutlet	Kotelett, Rippe
côtelette d'agneau	lamb cutlet	Lamm Kotelett
côtelette de mouton	mutton cutlet	Hammkotelett
cou	neck	Nacken
coulibiac	fishy patty	Fischpastete
coupe	cup	Schale
courge, potiron	pumpkin	Kürbis
courgette	vegetable marrow, courgette	Zucchetti, kleine Kurbisse
couteau	knife	Messer
couvert	cover (lay-up)	Gedeck
crabe	crab	Krabbe
crème	cream	Sahne
crème anglaise	custard	Eiercreme, englische Creme
crème d'avoine	cream of oatmeal	Haferschleimsuppe
crème de menthe	peppermint liqueur	Pfeffermünzlikör
crème fouettée	whipped cream	Schlagsahne
crème d'orge	barley soup	Gerstenschleim
crème de volaille	chicken cream soup	Geflügelcremesuppe
crème aux amandes	Almond cream	Mandelcreme
crêpes	pancakes	Pfannkuchen
crépinettes	flat sausages	Netzwürstchen
cresson	wattercress	Wasserkresse
crevettes	shrimps, prawns	Krabben
croquettes	fritters	Krusteln
croûte	crust	Kruste

French	English	German
cru	raw	roh
cruche	jug	Krug
cuillère	spoon	Löffel
cumin	carraway seed	Kümmel
cuire	cook, boil (to)	Kochen, sieden
cuisine	kitchen	Küche
cuisinier	cook	Koch
cuissot	haunch	Keule
cuit	cooked	gekocht
culinaire	culinary	Kochkunst
cure-dents	toothpick	Zahnstocher
curcuma	tumeric	Kurkuma
cygne	swan	Schwan

D

French	English	German
daim	deer	Dammhirsch
darne	fish steak	Fisch Steak
dattes	dates	Datteln
daube	stewed beef	geschmort
daurade	gold mackerel	Goldmakrele
débarrasser	clear away (to)	abräumen
déboucher	uncork (to)	entkorken
decanter	decant (to)	Abgießen, abfüllen
découper	carve, cut up (to)	zerlegen
déguster	taste, try (to)	kosten
délicatesse	delicacy	Delikatesse
démouler	remove the mould (to)	enthüllen, umstürzen
diable	devilled, devil style	Teufelsart
dinde	turkey	Puter
dindonneau	young turkey	Junger Truthahn
dîner	dinner	Abendessen, Diner
distillation	distillation	Destillation
dorade	sea bream	Goldbrassen
dorche	codling	Dorsch
douceur	sweetness	Süße
doux, douce	sweet	suß

French	English	German
E		
eau	water	Wasser
eau de source	spring water	Mineralwasser
eau-de-vie	brandy	Weinbrand
eau minérale	mineral water	Mineralwasser
ecorce	peel	Rinde, Schale
écraser	mash, squash (to)	zerdrücken
écrémer	cream (to)	abrahmen, entrahmen
écrevisse	crayfish	Krebs
écume	scum	Schaum
écumer	scum (to remove)	Abshäumen
émincé	sliced	Geschnetzeltes
en dés	diced	gewürfelt
encaver	cellar	einkellern
endives	chicory	Chicorée
entonnoir	funnel	Trichter
entrecôte	sirloin or entrecôte steak	Zwischenrippenstuuck
entremets	sweets, puddings	Süßspeise
épaule	shoulder	Schulter
épaule de mouton	shoulder of mutton	Hammelschulter
épaule de veau	veal shoulder	Kalbsschulter
éperlan	smelt	Stint
épi de maïs	corn on the cob	Maiskolben
épice	spice	Gewürz
épinard	spinach	Spinat
escalope	scallop	Schnitzel
escargot	snail	Schnecke
escarole	endive	Zichorie
estragon	tarragon	Estragon
esturgeon	sturgeon	Stör
étuvée	stewed	gedünstet
étuver	stew (to)	dünsten
évaporer	evaporate (to)	verdunsten
extrait, essence	essence	Auszug, Essenz

French	English	German
F		
facture	bill, the check	Rechnung
faîne	Beech nut	Bucheichel
faisan	pheasant	Fasan
farce	filling, stuffing	Füllunq
farci	stuffed, filled	gefüllt
farine	flour	Mehl
farineux	mealy, floury	Mehlig
fécule	starch flour	Stärkemehl
fenouil	fennel	Fenchel
féra	dace	Felchen
festin	banquet	Bankett
fête	festival	Fest
feuille	leaf	Blatt
fèves	broad beans	Dicke Bohnen
filet de boeuf	tenderloin, fillet of beef	Lendenstück
filets de sole	fillets of sole	Seezungenfilets
flamande	Flemish style	Flämische Art
flet	flounder	Flunder
flétan	halibut	Heilibutt
fleur	flower	Blume
fleurons	small puff pastry crescents	Fleurons, Blätterteighalbmonde
fleuriste	florist	Blumenhändler
flocon	flake	Flocke
fogas	fogash, pike perch	Fogasch, Fogas
foie	liver	Leber
foie de boeuf	beef liver	Rindsnieren
Foie gras	goose liver	Gänseleber
foncé	dark	dunkel
fondre	melt (to)	schmelzen
four	oven	Backofen
fourchette	fork	Gabel
frais	fresh, cool	frisch, kuhl
fraise	strawberry	Erdbeere
framboise	raspberry	Himbeere

French	English	German
fraper	beat, cool	schlagen, den Wein abkühlen
friandise	fancy biscuits, petit fours	Kleingebäch
fricandeau de veau	larded roast veal	Gespickter Kalbsbraten
fricasée de volaille	stewed chicken in white sauce	Weißes Geflügelragout
frire	fry, deep-fry (to)	frittieren
froid	cold	kalt
fromage	cheese	Käse
froment	wheat	Weizen
fruit	fruit	Obst
fruits séchés	dried fruits	Backobst
fumé	smoked	geräuchert
fumée	smoke	Rauch

G

French	English	German
gant	glove	Handschuh
garçon	waiter	Kellner, Ober
garde-manger	larder	Vorratsraum
garder	conserve, store (to)	aufbewahren
garniture	garnish	Garnierung, Garniture
gâteau	cake	Kuchen
gaufrette	wafer	Waffel
genièvre	juniper, gin	Wachholderbeere
gibier	game	Wild
gibier à plume	feathered game	Federwild
gibier à poil	furred game	Haarwild
gigot	hind led	Keule
gigot d'agneau	leg of lamb	Lammkeule
gigot de mouton	leg of mutton	Hammelkeule
gigue	leg of venison	Rekeule
gingembre	ginger	Ingwer
girofle	cloves	Gewürznelken
glace	ice	Eis
glace	Ice cream	Eiscreme
glacé	iced, frozen	gefroren
glacial	icy	eiskalt

French	English	German
glacière	ice-cellar	Eiskeller
gland	acorn	Eichel
gobelet	tumbler	Becher
goulache de boeuf	goulash	Rindsgulasch
goujon	gudgeon (small strips of sole)	Gründling
gourmand	gourmand	schlemmerhaft
gourmandise	delicatessen	Delicatesse
gourmet	connoisseur, gourmet	Feinschmecker
grand, gros	big, great, large, thick	Groß
gras, graisse	corn, grain	Korn, Getreide
gratin (au)	baked, crusted	überbacken
gratiner	bake, crust (to)	Im Ofen backen
grenade	pomegranate	Granatapfel
grenadin	scollops of veal	Kalbsschnitzel
grenadine	pomegranate syrop	Sirop Granatsaft
grenouille	frog	Frosch
gril	grill	Grill
grillé	grilled	gegrillt
grillade variée	mixed grill	gemischte Grillplatte
griottes	morello cherries	Sauerkirschen
grondin	gurnard	Knurrhahn
groseille noire, cassis	blackcurrant	schwarze Johannisbeere
groseille rouge	redcurrant	rote Johannisbeere
groseille vert	gooseberry	Stachelbeere
grouse	grouse	Waldhuhn
gruau	oatmeal, groats	Haferflecken

H

French	English	German
haché	minced	gehackt
hacher	hash, mince (to)	hacken, fein schneiden
hachis	hash	Hachfleisch
haricot	bean	Bohne
haricots blancs	white bean	weißeBohnen
haricots verts	French beans	grüne Bohnen
haricots noirs	black beans	schwarzeBohnen
hareng	herring	Hering

French	English	German
herbes	herbs	Kräuter
hiver	winter	Winter
homard	lobster	Hummer
hôte	guest, host	Gast
huile	oil	Öl
huitre	oyster	Auster

I

infusion	infusion, tea	Aufguss, Tee
infusion de camomille	camomile tea	Kamillentee
infusion de menthe	mint tea	Pfefferminztee
Infusion de tilleul	lime tea	Lindenblütentee

J

jambon	ham	Schinken
jardin	garden	Garten
jarret	knuckle	Haxe
jaune d'oeuf	egg yolk	Eigelb
jus, suc	juice, gravy	Saft

K

Kumquats, oranges naines	cumquats, dwarf oranges	Kumquats, Zwergorangen

L

lait	milk	Milch
laitue	lettuce	Kopfsalat
langoustine	Dublin bay prawn	Garnele
langue	tongue	Zunge
lapin	rabbit	Kaninchen
lapin de garenne	wild rabbit	Wildkaninchen
lard	bacon	Frühstücksspeck
lardé	larded	gespickt
lardoire	larding pin	Spicknadel

French	English	German
lardon	slice of bacon	Speckschnittchen
lasagnes	noodles	Bandnudeln
laurier	bay	Lorbeer
lavarret	sea trout	Seeforelle
légume	vegetable	Gemüse
lentilles	lentils	Linsen
levure	yeast	Hefe
liaison	combination, mixture	Verbindung, Mischung
lié	bound, thickened	legiert
lièvre	hare	Hase
lilas	lilac	Flieder
limande	lemon sole	Seezunge
limonade au citron	lemon squash	Zitronen limonade
liqueuer	liqueur	Likör
longe de veau	Loin of veal	Kalbsnierenbraten
lotte	eel	Aal
loup de mer	bass	Meerwolf

M

French	English	German
macaroni	maccaroni	Makkaroni
macédoine de fruits	fruit salad	Obstsalat
macérer	macerate (to)	ziehenlassen
mâche	corn salad, lambs lettuce	Feldsalat, Rapunzelsalat
maïs	maize	Mais
maître	master, householder	Meister, Hausherr/frau
maître d'hotel	head waiter	Oberkellner
malt	malt	Malz
mandarine	mandarine	Mandarine
manger	eat (to)	essen
maquereau	mackerel	Räucherhering
marcassin	young wild boar	Frischling
marchand de vin	wine merchant	Weinhändler
margarine	margarine	Margarine
marmelade	compote, marmalade	Marmelade
marmite	cooking pot	Kochtopf
mariné	pickles	eingelegt

French	English	German
marron	chestnut	Kastanie, Edelkastaine
massepain	marzipan	Marzipan
masquer	mask (to)	maskieren
médaillons de boeuf	medallions of beef	Rindsmedaillons
mélange	mixture	Mischung
mélanger	mix, blend (to)	mischen, vermischen
mêlé	mixed	gemischt
mêler	mix (to)	mischen
melon	melon	Melone
menthe	mint	Minze
menu	menu, bill o fare	Speisekarte
menu gastronomique	gastronomic menu	Feinschmeckermenü
menu de Noël	Christmas menu	Weinachtsmenu
menu de Pâques	Easter menu	Ostermenü
mer	sea	Meer, See
merlan	whiting	Weißling
mets	meal, food	Gericht, Speise
miel	honey	Honig
mignon, mignonne	little, small	niedlich, klein
mijoter	simmer (to)	Schmoren, langsam ziehen lassen
mirabelle	mirabelle, small yellow plum	Kleine gelbe Pflaume, Mirabelle
mode	fashion, style, method	Mode, Methode, Rübe
mollet	soft, tender	weich, zart
morceau	piece, part	Stück
morceler	mince, divide, cut (to)	zerteilen
morille	moril (mushroom)	Morchel
mortifer	tenderise meat (to)	Fleisch zart machen
morue	codfish	Kabeljau
moule	mussel	Muschel
moulin	mill	Mühle
moulu	milled, ground	gemahlen
mousse	foam	Schaum
mousseux	sparkling	schäumend
moût	must, grape juice	Most, Traubensaft
moutarde	mustard	Senf

French	English	German
mouton	mutton	Hammel
moyen, moyenne	middle-sized, average	Mittelgroß, durchschnittlich
mulet	mullet	Meerbarbe
mûr	ripe	reif
mûre	blackberry	Brombeere
muscade	nutmeg	Muskat
myrtille	blueberry	Heidelbeere

N

French	English	German
naturel	natural, genuine	natürlich, unverfälscht
navarin	mutton stew	Hammelragout
navet	turnip	Weiße Rübe
Noël	snow	Schnee
neige	Christmas	Weihnachten
noir	black	schwarz
noisette	hazelnut	Haselnuß
noix	nut	Nüss
noix du Brasil	Brazil nut	Paranuß
noix de coco	coconut	Kokosnuß
noix de veau	Loin of veal	Kalbsnuß
noix d'acajou	cashew nut	Acajou-Nüsse, Cashew-Nüsse, Flefantenlaus
note	account, bill	Rechnung
nouilles	noodles	Nudeln
noyau	kernel	Kern

O

French	English	German
odeur	odour, flavour	Geruch, Geschmack
oeuf	egg	Ei
oeuf à la coque	soft boiled egg	weichgekochtes Ei
oeufs brouilles	scrambled eggs	Rührei
oeuf en cocotte	eggs in cocotte	Eikoddler
oeuf frit	fried egg	Spiegelei
oeufs poché	poached eggs	Pochiertes Ei
oeufs à la neige	floating islands	Schnee-Eier

French	English	German
oeuf sur le plat	fried egg	Spiegeleier
oie	goose	Gans
oignon	onion	zwiebel
olives noirs	black olives	schwarze Oliven
omble chevalier	golden trout	Ritter, saibling
omelette	omelette	Eierkuchen
orange	orange	Apfelsine, Orange
orange amère	bitter orange	Bitterorange
orange sanguine	blood orange	Blutorange
orge	barley	Gerste
orge perlé	pearl barley	Rollgerste
origine	origin	Ursprung
oseille	sorrel	Sauerampfer
osso buco	knuckle of veal	Kalbshaxe
oursin	sea urchin	Seeigel

P

French	English	German
paille	straw, drinking straw	Stroh, Strohhalm
palée	ferra, trout	Bälchen, Felchen
palmier	palm tree	Palme
pamplemouse	grapefruit	Pampelmuse
pain	bread	Brot
pain d'épice	gingerbread	Lebkuchen
pain grilé	toast	Röstbrot
pain de seigle	rye bread	Roggenbrot
panaché	mixed	gemischt
pané	breadcrumbed	paniert
pannequet	pancake	Pfannkuchen
panier	basket	Korb
papier	paper	Papier
Pâques	Easter	Ostern
passoire	sieve	Sieb
Pastèque	Water melon	Wassermelone
pâte	paste, dough, batter	Teig
pâté	pie, pâté	Pastete
pâtisserie	pastry	Backware

French	English	German
pâtissier	pastry cook	Konditor
paupiettes de veau	rolled stuffed veal, veal olives	Roullade
pays	country	Land, Vaterland
paysan	country style	Bauernart
peau	skin	Haut
pêche	peach	Pfirsich
pelure	peel	Schale, Haut
pépin	kernel	Kern
perche	perch	Barsch
perdreau	partridge	Rebhuhn
persil	parsley	Petersilie
pesant	heavy in weight	schwer
petit	little, small	klein, unbedeutend
petit déjeuner	breakfast	Morgenessen
petit déjeuner américain	American breakfast	Amerikanisches Früstück
petit déjeuner continental	continental breakfast	kontinentales Früstück, Kontinentalfrüstück
petit déjeuner anglais	English breakfast	englisches Früstück
petit déjeuner rustique	farmer's breakfast	Bauernfrüstück
petit four	sweetmeats	kleines Geback
petit lait	buttermilk	Buttermilch
petit pois	green peas	grüne Erbsen
pied	foot	Fuß
pied de veau	calf's foot	Kalbsfuß
pigeon	pigeon	Taube
pigeon sauvage	wild pigeon	Wildtaube
piment	pimento	Pfeffer
pintade	guinea fowl	Perlhuhn
piquant	spicy	schart
piqué	larded	mit Speck gespickt
pissenlit	dandelion	Löwenzahn
pistache	pistachio	Pistazie
plat	dish	Gericht, Schüssel
plateau	tray	Tablett
plie, carrelet	plaice	Goldbutt
pointes d' asperges	asparagus tips	Spargelspitze
poire	pear	Birne

French	English	German
Poires William	William pears, bartlett pears	Williamsbirnen
poireau	leek	Porree
pois	peas	Erbse
pois frais	fresh peas	Frischerbsen
pois chiches	chick peas	Kichererbsen
pois mangetout	mangetout, snow peas	Zuchererbsen
poisson	fish	Fisch
poitrine	breast	Brust
poivre	pepper	Pfeffer
poivre de cayenne	cayenne pepper	Kayennepfeffer
poivron, piment	green or red pepper, pimento	Pfefferschote, Paprika
pommes de terre	apple	Apfel
pomme	potato	Kartoffel
porc	pork, pig	Schwein
porcelet	piglet, young pig	Ferkel, Jungschwein
porridge	porridge	Haferbrei
potage	soup	Suppe
potiron	pumpkin	Kürbis
pouding	pudding	Pudding
poularde	fattened pullet	Masthuhn
poulet	chicken	Huhn
poussin	spring chicken	Küiken
praliné	burnt almond	Gebrannte Mandel
pression	pressure, steam pressure	Druck, Dampfdruck
prix	price	Preis
propriétaire	proprietor, owner	Eigentümer
prune	plum	Pflaume
pruneau	prune	Zwetschge
pulpe	pulp	Fruchtfleisch, Gemüsefleisch
pur	pure, clear	rein
purée	mash, purée	Mus
purée de pommes	apple purée	Apfelmus
purée de pommes de terre	mashed potatoes	Kartoffelbrei
Purée de pois	mashed peas	Erbsenbrei

French	English	German
Q		
Queue	tail	Schwanz
Queue de boeuf	oxtail	Ochsenschwanz
Quenelle	dumpling, ball	Klöße, Knödel
Quenelles de foie gras	goose liver dumplings	Gänseleberklößchen
R		
râble de lievre	saddle of hare	Hasenrücken
racine	root	Wurzel
racler	shave, scrape (to)	schaben, raspeln
radis	radishes	Radieschen
raffiner	refine (to)	verfeinern
rafraîchir	cool, refresh (to)	abkühlen, erfrischen
ragoût	stew, ragout	Würzfleisch, Ragout
raie	skate	Rochen
raifort	horseradish	Meerrettich
raisin	grape	Weintraube
raisins de corinthe	currant, raisins	Rosinen
raisins de marc	redcurrants	Johanisbeeren
râpé	grated	gerieben
rave	root	wurzel
ravioli au foie gras	goose-liver ravioli	Gänselleberravioli
recette	receipt, recipe	Einnahme
réchaud	hotplate	Wärmeplatte
réchauffer	warm up (to)	aufwärmen
recuit	cooked again	wiedergekocht
récurer	scour, clean (to)	scheuern, reinigen
refroidir	refresh, cool (to)	abkülen
refroidissement	cooling	Erkalten
reine-claude	greengages	Königspflaume
repas	meal	Mahlzeit
requin	shark	Haifisch
rhubarbe	rhubarb	Rhabarber
riche	rich	schwer
rince-doigts	fingerbowl	Fingerschale

French	English	German
rincer	rinse (to)	spülen
ris de veau	sweetbread	Kalbs Bries
rivière	river	Fluß
riz	rice	Reis
rognon	kidney	Niere
rognon de boeuf	beef kidney	Rindsnieren
roi	king	König
romarin	rosemary	Rosmarin
rôti, le rôti	roasted, roast	gebraten, Braten
rôti à la broche	roasted on spit	am Spieß Gebraten
rouget	red mullet	Rot barsch
rumpsteak	rump steak	Rumpsteak

S

French	English	German
safran	saffron	Safran
sagou	sago	Sago
saignant	underdone	blutig, bleu
saindoux	pork dripping, lard	Schweinefett, Schmalz
saison	season	Jahreszeit
salade	salad	Salat
salade, mâche, doucette	corn salad	Feldsalat
salade de fruits	fruit salad	Obst salat
saler	salt (to)	salzen
salle à manger	dining room	Speisesaal
salsifis, scorsonères	salsify, oyster plant	Schwarzwurzeln
sandre	perch pike	Zander, Hechtbarsch
sandwich	sandwich	belegtes Brot
sang	blood	Blut
sanglier	wild boar	Wildschwein
santé	health	Gesundheit
sardine	sardine	Sardine
sauce	sauce, gravy	Sauce, Soße
sauce à l'estragon	tarragon sauce	Estragonsauce
sauce au pain anglaise	bread sauce	englische Brotsauce
saucisse	sausage	Würstchen
saucisson	sausage	Wurst

French	English	German
sauge	sage	Salbei
saumon	salmon	Lachs
sauté	sautéed	sautiert
sauvage	wild	wild
sec	dry	trocken, herb
sel, salière	salt, salt cellar	Salz, salzstreuer
selle	saddle	Rücken
selle de chevreuil	saddle of venison	Rehrücken
semoule	semolina	Gries
séparer	separate (to)	Trennen, teilen
serviette	napkin	Serviette
sirop	syrup	Sirup
sole	sole	Seezunge
sommelier	wine waiter, wine butler	Wein Kellner, Ober
soubis	mashed onion	Zwiebelmus
soucoupe	saucer	Untertasse
soufflé	soufflé	Auflauf
soupe	soup	Suppe
soupe froide	cold soup	kaltschale
souper	supper	Abendessen
soupière	soup tureen	Suppenschlüssel
source	spring	Quelle, Ursprung
suc	juice, sap	Saft
succulent	juicy	saftig
sucre	sugar	Zucker
sucre en poudre	castor sugar	puderzucker
sucre	sweetened	gezuckert
surprise	surprise	Uberaschung

T

French	English	German
table	table	Tisch, Tafel
table d'hôte	table d'hôte/set meal	Das Menü
tamis	sieve, sifter	Drahtsieb
tapioca	tapioca	Sagou
tarte	fruit tart	Obstkuchen
tartelette	tartlet	Törtchen

French	English	German
tartine	slice of buttered bread	Butterbrot
tartare	tartar, cream of tartar	Tartar
tasse	cup	Tasse, Schala
teint	colour	Farbe, Gesichtsfarbe
tendre	tender, soft	weich, zart
terre	earth	Erde
tête	head	Kopf
tête de veau	calf's head	Kalbskopf
thé	tea	Tee
théière	teapot	Teekanne
thon	tunny fish	Thunyfisch
thym	thyme	Thymian
tilleul	lime tea, lime infusion	Lindenblütentee
tire-bouchon	corkscrew	Korkenzieher
tisane	herbal tea, infusion	Gesundheitstee
tomate	tomato	Tomate
tonique	tonic, restorative	Stärkendes Mittel, Tonikum
tonneau	vat, barrel	Faß, Tonne
topinambour	Jerusalem artichoke	Artischoke
tortue	turtle	Schildkröte
tourte	cake, tart	Torte
traiteur	caterer	Stadtlieferant für Speisen
tranche	slice	Schnitte, Scheibe
trancheur	cut, carve (to)	schneiden
tranchoir	cutting-board	Schneide brett
transvaser	decant (to)	Umgießen, abgießen
tremper	soak (to)	einweichen
trier	select, pick out (to)	auslesen
tripes	tripes	Pansen
truffe	truffle	Trüffel
truite	trout	Forelle
truite saumonée	Salmon trout	Lachsforelle
tulipe	tulip	Tulpe
turbot	turbot	Steinbutt

French	English	German
V		
vache	cow	Kuh
vanille	vanilla	Vanille
vapeur	steam, vapour	Dampf
veau	veal, calf	Kalb
végétal	vegetable	Pfanzlich
velouté	cream soup	Sahnesuppe, Cremesuppe
vendange	vintage	Weinlese, Ernte
verdure	vegetables, greenery	Gemüse, Grünes
verger	orchard	Obstgarten
vermicelles	vermicelli	Fadennudeln
vert	green	grün
viande	meat	Fleisch
vieux	old	alt
vigne	vine	Weinstock
vigneronne	wine grower's style	Winzerart
vignoble	vineyard	Weinbau
vin	wine	Wein
vin mousseux	sparkling wine	Schaumwein, Sekt
vinaigre	vinegar	Essig
viticulture	wine growing	Weinberg, Weingegend
vol-au-vent	vol-au-vent, puff pastry pie	Blätterteigpastete
volaille	poultry, chicken	Geflügel